K. R. Karsch, K. K. Haase (Eds.)

Coronary Laser Angioplasty

An Update

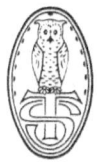

Springer-Verlag Berlin Heidelberg GmbH

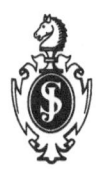

The Editors:
Prof. Dr. K. R. Karsch
Dr. K. K. Haase
Medizinische Klinik III
Abteilung Kardiologie
Otfried-Müller-Straße
7400 Tübingen

Die Deutsche Bibliothek – CIP-Einheitsaufnahme

Coronary laser angioplasty: an update / K. R. Karsch; K. K.
Haase (Hrsg.).
   ISBN 978-3-662-06418-4   ISBN 978-3-662-06416-0 (eBook)
   DOI 10.1007/978-3-662-06416-0
NE: Karsch, Karl–Rüdiger [Hrsg.]

Copyright © 1991 by Springer-Verlag Berlin Heidelberg
Originally published by Dr. Dietrich Steinkopff Verlag GmbH & Co. KG, Darmstadt in 1991
Softcover reprint of the hardcover 1st edition 1991
Medical Editorial: Sabine Müller — English Editor: James C. Willis — Production: Heinz J.
Schäfer

Printed on acid-free paper

Preface

Since the development of the first laser generator by Maiman in 1960, laser energy has gained increased interest and has subsequently been used in various fields of application. Due to its high energy density, combined with a sharply defined irradiation field, laser has aroused great expectations, especially since laser beams have been used very successfully in various fields especially technology and medicine.

Medical and surgical applications of the laser were among the first and have been of undisputed benefit in, for example, ophthalmologic interventions such as coagulation of the retina, or for endoscopic tumorectomy in the bronchial, gastrointestinal and urogenital tracts.

Consequently, considerable research effort was made to also apply laser techniques in interventional cardiology for the treatment of atherosclerosis, aimed at removing plaque material from stenosed tissue or occluded ateries and recanalizing tough and calcified segments unsuitable for the well-extablished technique of balloon dilatation. Ablating atheroma rather than pushing it aside was thought to achieve better results. However, it was found that the laser may create rough-edged cuts partly with substantial thermal or mechanical damage to the surrounding tissue, consequently provoking preconditions for unwanted restenosis.

Different types of laser generators and probes have therefore been investigated in arterial vessels, mostly focusing on indirect laser effects. Intravasal probes with laser-heated metal tips were used, as well as balloon catheters with an incorporated laser fiber designed to heat the surrounding tissue outside the balloon and to, ineffect, "iron out the plaque".

However, it has been demonstrated that the application of thermal lasers has gained no advantage over the wellestablished therapeutic procedures. There are, on the other hand, also less demanding techniques such as those employing high-frequency currents to achieve local heating.

Considering general principles and the in vitro results it has appeared more suitable to use the photoablative qualities of the excimer laser. High-frequency laser energies and their electric fields are capable of forcing electrons out of the atomic bond, thus breaking the molecular compound with minimal damage to the surrounding tissue. Moreover, there is virtually no risk of peripheral embolism on account of the very small size of the debris.

When the initial technical difficulties with the transmission of this energy through appropriate probes had been overcome, the invention of the excimer laser launched clinical investigations in many centers, the results of which are being communicated here.

With the excimer laser it is possible to pass short and though stenoses which cannot be dilated using balloon catheters, for example, in the case of a stenosed aortic orifice. In most cases, however, an additional balloon dilatation is indicated. Also, entertaining the hope that this technique might help to reduce the restenosis rate does not seem justified. Finally, applying excimer laser in the case of total occlusions has no advantage since the probe has to be guided along a wire, thus requiring a previous introduction and passing of a guidewire.

New technical developments are being highlighted, for example, the holmium laser. It has also appeared promising to use bundled energy beams in the ultraviolet rang with the supposition that they activate certain proliferation-inhibiting substances in the tissue.

For the time being, the results of laser intervention have to be compared to those of balloon dilatation. More than 10 years of experience with balloon angioplasty have revealed that good long-term results can be achieved in most cases. Any restenosis (rate: 25–30%) can usually be redilatated, leading to a restenosis rate of less than 10%.

It appears that laser-assisted removal of atheromatous material has no advantage in regard to the restenosis rate. This consequence is also in line with the experience gained in surgical endatherectomy and directional catheter atherectomy. It might even be said that the more material comprising the media that is ablated, the higher the risk for restenosis. A similar effect may also occur following thermal tissue damage caused by a laser balloon.

This book presents an in-depth, comprehensive review of the state of laser techniques in coronary artery stenosis. It is recommended to anyone concerned with either clinical laser application or basic research.

Frankfurt, June 1991   M. Kaltenbach

Foreword

This book is aimed at informing cardiologists involved experimentally or clinically in studies of reduction of atherosclerotic plaque in coronary arteries. The more sophisticated a method, the higher the individual expectations. However, every new method for the treatment of disabling disease has to be evaluated carefully and compared to current medical standards in regard to efficacy and complications.

It is our sincere belief that early statements regarding the efficacy of a new method have to be postponed until the new technique attains standards comparable to current techniques.

To encourage rational development and further discussion, insight into the individual method has to be broadened and the current "state of the art" has to be defined.

Tübingen, June 1991   The editors

Contents

Lasers for Angioplasty

E. Steiger

E. Steiger Lasertechnik GmbH, Gröbenzell, FRG

Introduction

In 1917, Einstein theoretically predicted a quantum phenomena called laser (acronym for *Light Amplification by Stimulated Emission of Radiation*).

It was not until 1958 that Schawlow and Townes first described the conditions for laser action at optical frequencies, and finally, in 1960, the first demonstration of laser action by Maiman was achieved using ruby (chromium-doped sapphire), a crystalline solid system, as amplification or gain medium.

Parallel to this, Gould invented the gas laser. Spin-offs of this idea were the realization of the CO_2-laser by Patel, and the argon, krypton, and xenon lasers by Gordon and co-workers in 1964. Also in 1964, Geusic and co-workers explored Nd:YAG (neodymium-doped yttrium aluminum garnet), a crystal that soon achieved a position of dominance among solid-state laser materials because it is very hard, has a good thermal conductivity, can be grown and fabricated in a manner that yields laser rods with high optical quality, and permits laser operation at high average power levels. It is still a "work-horse" in many medical and surgical applications of lasers that started in 1962 with Goldman's first use of the ruby laser in dermatology.

Since then, a tremendous research effort has continued in many medical specialities, including in cardiovascular and peripheral artery disease.

But it was not until 1980 that Macruz published results of the ablation of arteriosclerotic plaque with a continuous wave (cw) argon-ion laser, and Choy described a laser catheter for recanalizing arterial obstructive lesions.

In 1983, Ginsburg was the first to recanalize an occluded artery in a human patient, and later the same year, Choy and colleagues performed successful argon laser recanalization of coronary arteries in five human patients during coronary bypass graft surgery.

Two years later, Coy et al. performed percutaneous laser recanalization of carotid arteries in man, and Cumberland and Sanborn used a "hot-tip catheter" — a metal tip at the distal end of a fiberoptic delivery system heated by an argon-ion laser beam — to recanalize stenotic femoral arteries, prior to conventional balloon angioplasty. This technique, however, in which also cw Nd:YAG laser sources were used to heat the tip, is not a true laser-recanalization since there is no direct laser/plaque-interaction. Later, modified fiberoptic tips, such as sapphire tips, combined metal cap/sapphire tips, or lensed tips were used together with cw argon-ion and Nd:YAG lasers to study the combined effects of heat and direct laser irradiation. Nevertheless, cw laser radiation produced charring or thermal injury to the residual irradiated arterial surface, and bare fibers showed a high risk of perforation due to the small bending radii of the involved vessels, mainly in coronary arteries.

Beginning in 1984, pulsed laser systems for direct plaque ablation gained increased interest, because pulsed laser energy eliminated nearly all gross, light microscopic, and ultrastructural signs of thermal injury. Nearly identical results were obtained using the three harmonics of the Nd:YAG laser (355, 532, and 1064 nm), the pulsed CO_2 laser (TEA laser), or the excimer laser, if the energy dosis was carefully adjusted according to the wavelength of the laser emission. The most extensively studied system so far is the excimer laser at wavelengths of 308 and 351 nm, together with multifiber laser catheters as lightguides for laser angioplasty in coronary and peripheral arteries [6–8, 17–19, 23, 27, 28].

Recently, some other pulsed laser systems have emerged to compete with the excimer laser in angioplasty: solid-state lasers like the Ho:YAG, Tm:YAG, Er:YAG, or the frequency-doubled alexandrite laser, as they are more reliable, easier to handle, do not use toxic gases, and can be constructed as compact units that better fit the clinical environment. Also, flashlamp-pumped, pulsed, dye lasers with adjustable wavelengths in the region of 400–700 nm are currently under investigation [5, 11, 14, 22, 31, 33].

All the above systems have different wavelengths, pulse durations, and pulse shapes. How important such laser parameters can be for plaque ablation will be discussed in detail in the following.

Importance of different laser parameters

No matter what type of amplification medium is used for the generation of coherent and monochromatic laser light, either solid, liquid, or gas, all laser systems operate by the same physical process of stimulated emission of radiation. Figure 1 shows schematically the laser resonator or laser cavity that consists of an active or gain medium enclosed in a set of reflection mirrors. The gain medium is pumped by an external energy source (radiation, current, particles) that is controlled by an electronic circuit which

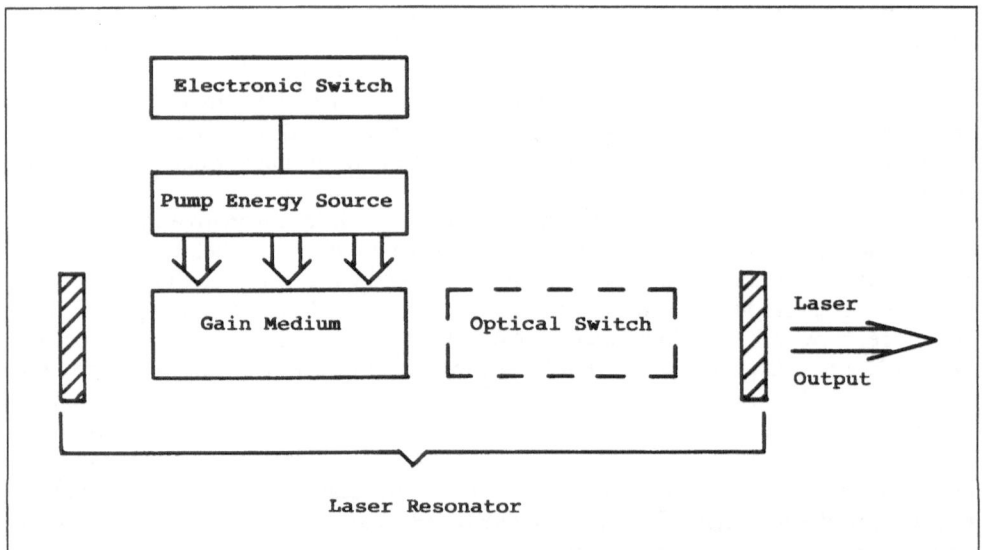

Fig. 1. Schematic of an optical laser resonator.

Table 1. Survey of characteristic laser parameters.

Wavelength
Pulse duration
Temporal pulse shape
Pulse energy
Repetition rate
Radial intensity distribution
Beam divergence

is responsible for the duration of the pump-pulse (cw or pulsed) to the active medium. Within the laser resonator the light emitted from the gain medium bounces back and forth between the mirrors tuned for resonance, stimulating more light emission from the active medium. One of the mirrors of the laser cavity normally is totally reflecting; the second mirror reflects the light of the gain medium only partially, allowing some of the laser light to exit the resonator. An optional optical switch inside or outside the laser cavity can further considerably reduce the pulse duration of the laser output (which is determined by the electronic switch duration, characteristics of the atoms and molecules of the gain medium, and the physical length of the resonator).

The laser output beam that exits the laser cavity is always characterized by its individual parameters, including wavelength, pulse duration, temporal pulse shape, pulse energy, repetition rate, radial intensity distribution, and beam divergence (Table 1). These features strongly determine the interaction of the laser beam with tissue, especially atherosclerotic diseased vessel tissue, whether it is of yellow atheromatous, fibrous, or calcified structure. Tissue characteristics like reflection and absorption coefficients, thermal conductivity, density, heat capacity, heat of vaporization, and melting temperature are responsible for the behavior of the biological material irradiated by the particular laser source.

To get a better insight into the complex laser beam/tissue-interaction it is worth looking at some special laser-beam properties in combination with tissue ablation during angioplastic procedures.

Laser wavelength

Of particular importance in laser/tissue-interaction is a search for a laser wavelength that is highly absorbed by plaque material, but only barely absorbed by healthy vascular tissue. Such a wavelength would permit an effective destruction of the diseased part, and minimize the damage to the healthy arterial wall.

Figure 2 shows the well-known absorption curve of water together with the measured absorption coefficient of soft tissue material with a water content of 60% vs wavelength in a wide spectral range of 0.1–10 µm. Three regions can be easily distinguished: In the wavelength range of approx. 300 to about 1300 nm the water absorption can be neglected; tissue absorption is also low, but orders of magnitudes higher than for water alone. This is due to the tissue chromophores like hemoglobin which peaks around 415, 540, and 577 nm. For wavelengths between 620 and 800 nm there is little absorption by blood – especially around 670 nm – but still a reasonable absorption by plaque exists [12].

3

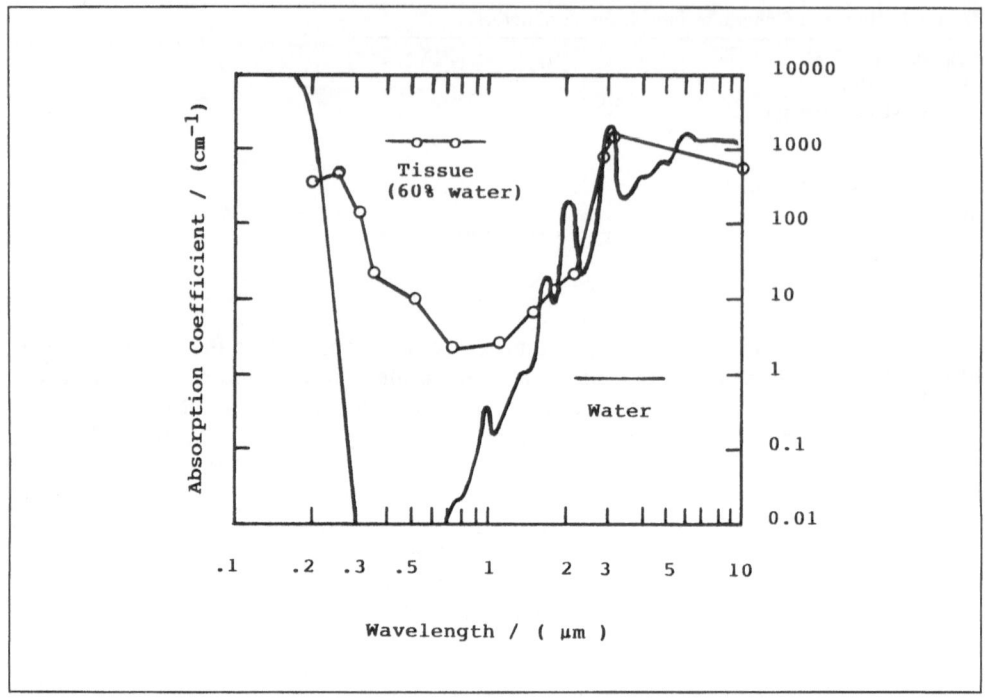

Fig. 2. Absorption coefficient of water and soft tissue with 60% water content vs wavelength.

In the wavelength region beyond approx. 1.5 μm, tissue absorption is mainly dominated by its water content. At a wavelength of more than about 3 μm the laser/tissue-interaction is independent of the tissue composition.

In the UV range of 250–290 nm the absorption coefficient of tissue is governed by protein absorption (aromatic amino acids and DNA). Below 200 nm water is again the dominant absorber, so that similar laser/tissue-effects can be expected for wavelengths longer than 3 μm or shorter than 200 nm.

Looking at the photon energies of different laser sources clearly indicates that in a simple one-photon absorption process more than 4 eV are necessary for the direct bond-breaking of a $C-C$ bond, and more than 6 eV for a $C=C$ bond (Table 2).

Regarding atherosclerotic tissue, it was found that atheromas absorb more than normal aorta, i. e., between 420 and 530 nm. In this wavelength range the average atheroma absorption due to yellow chromophores (consisting predominantly of a mixture of carotenoids) is more than 1.7 times that of a normal artery. A comparison of the beta carotene absorption spectra with the lipophilic chromophores extracted from atheroma suggests that some of the extract could be beta carotene, a known component of atherosclerotic lesions [26]. Microspectral photometry of arteries of the elastic type (Aorta abdominalis) and the muscular type (Arteria femoralis communis) revealed absorption peaks at 285 and 290 nm, respectively. The extinction of endothelium and muscle is most pronounced, while that of the subendothelial deposit is less pronounced. Laser wavelengths around 300 nm are mainly absorbed by the intima, media, and adven-

Table 2. Survey of the different types of bond-breaking in a one-photon-process vs laser wavelength.

Laser system	Laser wavelength (nm)	Photon energy (eV)	Type of direct bond-breaking (1-photon-process)
CO_2	10 600	0.12	–
Nd:YAG (f)	1 064	1.16	–
Alexandrite (f)	720–860	1.44–1.72	Si−Si
Nd:YAG (2f)	532	2.33	Si−Si
Dye (f)	400–700	1.77–3.10	S−S
Excimer (XeF)	352	3.53	C−N
			C−Br
Excimer (XeCl)	308	4.02	Br−H
			C−O
			C−C
			C−Cl
Excimer (KrF)	248	5.00	O−H
			H−H
			H−Cl
			C−H
Excimer (ArF)	193	6.42	Si−F
			F−H
			O−O
			C=C

(f = fundamental; 2f = frequency-doubled)

titia. The intermediate layers, especially atherosclerotic connective tissue, contribute little to absorption [13].

In order to enhance selective tissue ablation during angioplastic procedures, artificial chromophores like sudan black, cardiogreen, hematoporphyrin derivative, or tetracycline have been used. Intravenous administration of tetracycline in patients undergoing vascular surgery showed an enhanced ultraviolet laser ablation of tetracycline-treated atheroma compared to untreated atheroma, due to a pronounced absorption peak of tetracycline at 355 nm. This peak is absent in both treated and untreated normal vessel wall [24, 27].

Laser pulse duration

With the aid of electronic modules and/or optical components, gas, liquid, or solid-state lasers can produce pulselengths in an extremely large timescale, ranging from cw to femtosecond duration. Operating a cw-laser in a so-called chopped-mode, pulse durations in the second to millisecond range can be produced. In the "pulsed"-mode, durations in the millisecond to microsecond range; in the "Q-switched"-mode, in the microsecond to nanosecond range, and in the "mode-locked"-mode of operation, picosecond to femtosecond durations can be reached. The shorter the pulselength, the higher the laser peak power (Fig. 3), which leads to different and complex laser/tissue-interactions in using such laser pulses for removing diseased vascular tissue. Herein, pulse duration is directly correlated to thermal and acoustic injury of vessel wall structures.

5

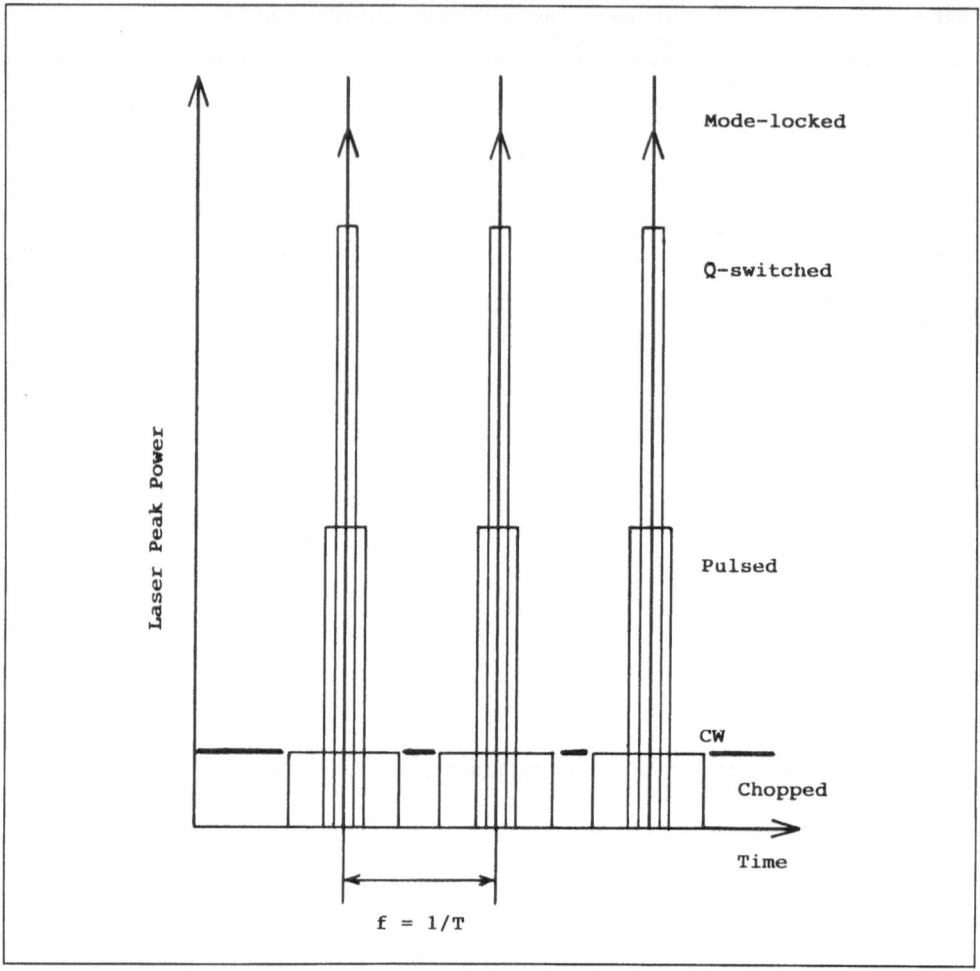

Fig. 3. Schematic of the laser peak power obtainable by cw; chopped; pulsed; Q-switched, and mode-locked lasers.

Thermal effects have been found mainly in using cw or chopped lasers like the argon-ion or the Nd:YAG laser. At high peak power levels of the laser pulse thermal pyrolisis is produced which results in direct vaporization of the irradiated tissue. At extremely high peak power levels nonlinear effects such as photodecomposition or photoablation (an effect described later in detail) occurs.

At even higher power levels a physical process called "optical breakdown" is induced, which results in a mechanical disruption of the affected tissue by acoustic shock waves [23]. To trigger that process, an ionized gas or plasma must be created in the surrounding liquid of the plaque material (either blood or saline solution), or in the diseased tissue itself. Within the total laser pulse duration (in the case of a Q-switched laser, on the order of 5–800 ns) a plasma is formed by multiphoton ionization in which the free electrons are accelerated in the laser radiation field by a process called "inverse bremsstrahlung'', causing a multiplication of the electrons by colliding with atoms and molecules of the medium. The remaining pulse energy not triggering the plasma process is scattered and absorbed, thus heating the plasma, which expands, driving a shock front with a velocity several times the speed of sound into the medium. The cooling plasma bubble leaves a cavity which expands against the static pressure of the liquid surrounding the plasma until a maximum radius is reached. The bubble then collapses and further oscillates with smaller radii, until it fully dissipates.

Figure 4 shows a laser-induced optical breakdown by a Q-switched, frequency-doubled Nd:YAG laser with a pulse duration of 8 ns in a trough with degassed water, used to study shock wave formation and propagation. The laser beam enters the trough from below and is focused by an optical lens inside the water. At the time of optical breakdown a plasma is induced by the high peak power laser beam. It can be seen that not all of the green laser radiation is absorbed, but instead a considerable amount is transmitted through the plasma.

The temporal shapes of such created shock waves are completely different for a Q-switched Nd:YAG laser with only 10 ns pulsewidth in comparison to a flashlamp-pumped pulsed dye laser with a pulse duration of 1 μs (Fig. 5). The solid-state laser pressure curve reveals a very fast risetime of the shock-wave front, within a few tens of ns timescale, whereas the liquid laser produces a much slower rise with even a slower decrease. The pressure transducer used for both laser systems indicates a peak pressure amplitude of about 640 bar, with only 90 mJ pulse energy of the Nd:YAG laser, and 320 bar with 800 mJ pulse energy of the dye laser.

Summarizing our experimental results and the results of other groups, it could be found that the peak pressure produced by laser-induced optical breakdown is indirect proportional to the distance from the breakdown, directly proportional to the square root of the laser pulse energy, indirectly proportional to the square root of the rise time of the shock wave pulse, and also indirectly proportional to the square root of the propagation velocity of the shock wave in the medium.

In order to maintain the necessary specificity of localized laser-interaction with minimal thermal injury, the laser pulsewidth must be carefully chosen to avoid degrading the

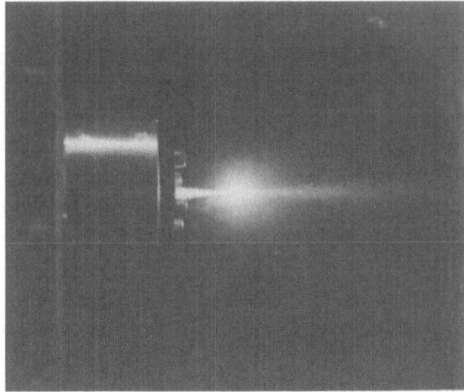

Fig. 4. Laser-induced optical breakdown by a Q-switched, frequency-doubled, Nd:YAG laser in water ($t_p = 8$ ns, $E_p/300$ mJ).

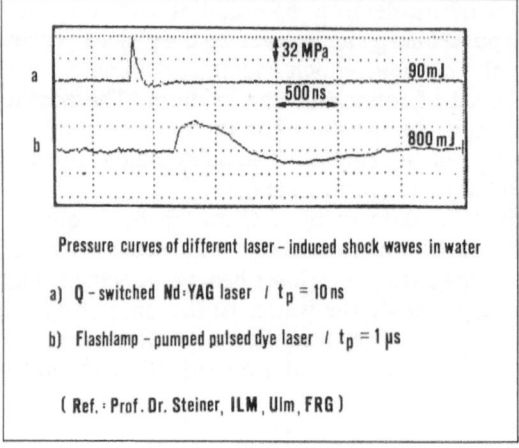

Pressure curves of different laser - induced shock waves in water

a) Q - switched Nd:YAG laser / t_p = 10 ns

b) Flashlamp - pumped pulsed dye laser / t_p = 1 μs

(Ref. : Prof. Dr. Steiner, ILM, Ulm, FRG)

Fig. 5. Temporal shape of the acoustic transients of laser-induced shock waves in water by a Q-switched Nd:YAG, and a flashlamp-pumped, pulsed dye laser.

Table 3. Tissue absorption coefficient and critical time-constant for laser/tissue-interaction vs laser wavelength.

Laser system	Laser wavelength (nm)	α in tissue (cm^{-1})	t_p (μsec)
CO$_2$	10 600	600	514
Er:YAG	2 940	2 700–4 500	9–25
Ho:Tm:Er:YAG	2 060	35	1.5×10^5
Er:YLF	1 730	15	8×10^5
Nd:YAG (f)	1 064	4	1×10^7
Ruby	694.3	5	7×10^6
Nd:YAG (2f)	532	12	1×10^6
Excimer (XeF)	351	40	1×10^5
Excimer (XeCl)	308	200	4 629
Excimer (KrF)	248	600	514
Excimer (ArF)	193	>400	<1 157

(f = fundamental; 2f = frequency-doubled)

sharpness and precision made possible by a high absorption coefficient of tissue for special wavelengths regions. Therefore, heat must not diffuse any distance greater than the penetration depth into tissue, which is given by the reciprocal of the absorption coefficient α. The maximum pulsewidth (t_p) a laser should have is therefore proportional to $(k\alpha^2)^{-1}$, where k is the thermal diffusivity of biological tissue, which is about 0.0012–0.0015 cm^2 s^{-1}. Table 3 gives this critical time-constant for some common laser systems in microseconds, together with the tissue absorption coefficient α for 60% water content. Except for the Er:YAG laser (λ=2940 nm, t_p=9–25 μs) and the CO$_2$ laser (λ=10 600 nm, t_p=514 μs) all other systems mentioned can have non-critical possible pulsewidths, even the four excimer laser lines. In reality, however, many conditions can modify this basic approximation for the thermal ablation by lasers, because convective currents may increase thermal loss from the target (particularly in a wet field) for longer pulse durations or repetitive pulses. For hard tissue, such as calcified plaque, thermal ablation may be a less efficient or even an ineffective method of tissue removal if the force generated by vaporization of tissue water is not able to disrupt the calcified structures. On the other hand, the effects of shock waves generated by short, high peak power pulses and high tissue absorption coefficients may increase ablation efficiency, particularly for calcified plaque [4, 11].

Laser pulse energy and repetition rate

When a pulsed or Q-switched laser beam is focused by an optical lens on a small spot or transmitted via optical fibers with core diameters of 200–400 µm, a very high laser intensity or fluence is created at the focal spot or at the distal end of the fiber. When tissue is irradiated under such conditions, a typical photoablation curve (as drawn in Fig. 6) is normally obtained when the ablation rate of the material is drawn vs fluence or laser pulse energy at a constant spot-size area.

Three different regions A, B, and C can be distinguished with a specific ablation threshold intensity $I_{threshold}$ that is dependent on the wavelength and absorption coefficients of the tissue material. Srinivasan and co-workers first described this effect when studying the ablation of synthetic organic polymers with an excimer laser at 193 nm and a pulse duration of 16 ns; they called this physical process, "ablative

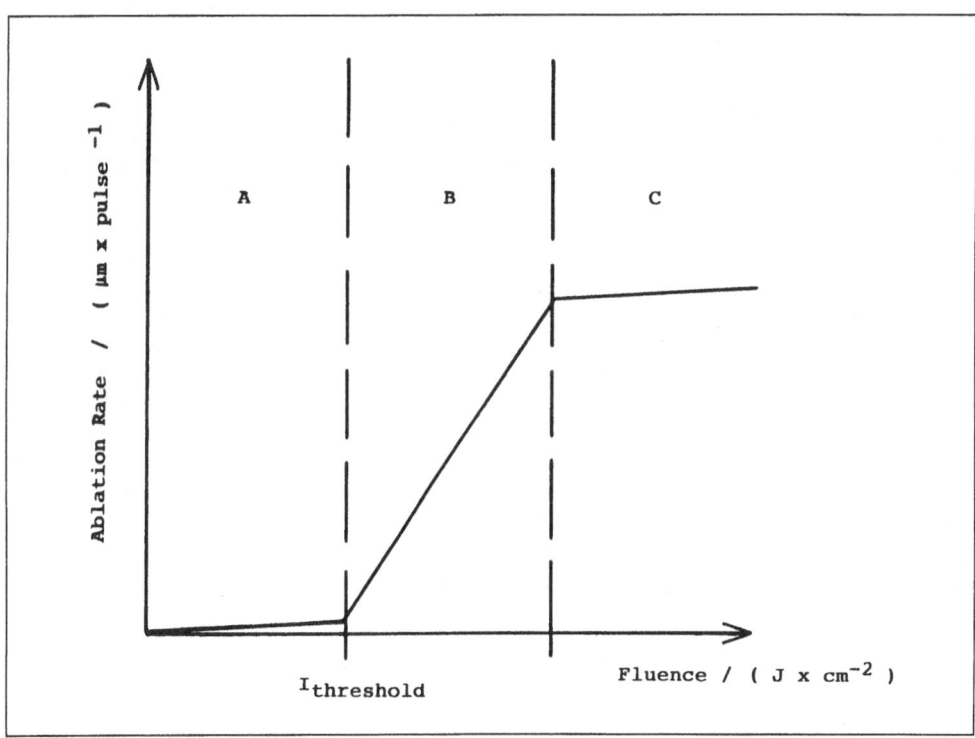

Fig. 6. Comparison of the ablation rate of tissue material vs fluence.

photodecomposition'' [29]. It is, however, still not exactly defined regarding what part of the process is induced by thermal removal of material, or by a break-up of molecular bonds (see Table 2).

In the nonablative regime (Region A), i. e., at a fluence below that of significant material removal, tissue is thermally heated. Acoustic transients measured with a piezoelectric film transducer attached to the tissue, consist of a compressive stress-wave generated by rapid heating, and thermal expansion of the sample surface related to the thermomechanical and optical properties of the tissue material. In this thermoelastic regime the stress is linearly related to the laser fluence if the pulse shape of the laser remains unchanged. However, with the inception of ablation at $I_{threshold}$, the efficiency of material removal increases rapidly (Region B). Whereas in the low fluence range the absorptivity of the tissue material for a given wavelength is independent of the fluence, the absorption instantaneously rises to near unity as the laser intensity at the surface of the sample approaches $I_{threshold}$ (anomalous absorption). The onset of the intensity-dependent absorption is always accompanied by a laser-induced plasma in the surface area. Also, the transient stress signal changes its shape significantly due to the recoil momentum transferred to the surface by ablation products. Within a definite pulse-energy regime, the ablation zone B, the ablation rate vs fluence shows a linear behavior until it reaches saturation (Region C). This is due to a plasma shielding effect which is not present in region B of the photoablation curve, since the opaque plasma in that region improves the energy coupling into tissue material.

With increasing fluences, however, the degree of ionization of the plasma is also increased, and the attenuation of the incident laser radiation grows. The plasma finally detaches from the tissue surface, expanding towards the origin of the laser beam. As a result, vaporization and, consequently, material removal are interrupted. As the plasma plume propagates back towards the laser, plasma heating decreases, the plasma becomes transparent, and the process starts again [10, 16].

In experimental work little difference in the ablation thresholds for normal and atheromatous tissue was found at wavelengths of 248, 308, and 532 nm with pulse durations of 10–15 ns [25]. Thus, it is very unlikely that a distinction between diseased and healthy tissue can be made by measuring and interpreting acoustic transients from tissue ablation in angioplastic procedures. However, there is strong evidence that the UV laser threshold for tissue ablation depends precisely on how many pulses are delivered to the sample, and at what pulse repetition rate of the laser system this is done. True, singleshot ablation thresholds would be higher than those achieved by repeated pulses. A high repetition rate of the laser system is also accompanied by an increased thermal load of the tissue material (even for the excimer laser lines) which result in higher thermal injury.

With an excimer laser at a wavelength of 308 nm, 17 ns pulse duration, fluences ranging from 0.3 to 3 J cm^{-2}, and repetition rates from 1 to 170 Hz, it was found that the removal rate of tissue is frequency-dependent, with varying degrees of thermal and mechanical injuries. The overall data indicate that it is preferable to enhance the repetition frequency of the ablation-laser than to enhance pulse energy when working in region B of the ablation curve [21].

Figure 7 also clearly indicates that the ablation threshold, $I_{threshold}$, is extremely wavelength-dependent, as shown for the wavelength region of 200 to 1100 nm. The material used for these experiments was tissue taken from the aorta abdominalis. Data collected for that ablation threshold curve come from pulsed and Q-switched lasers (excimer, Nd:YAG, and alexandrite) with pulse durations in the range of 10 to

10

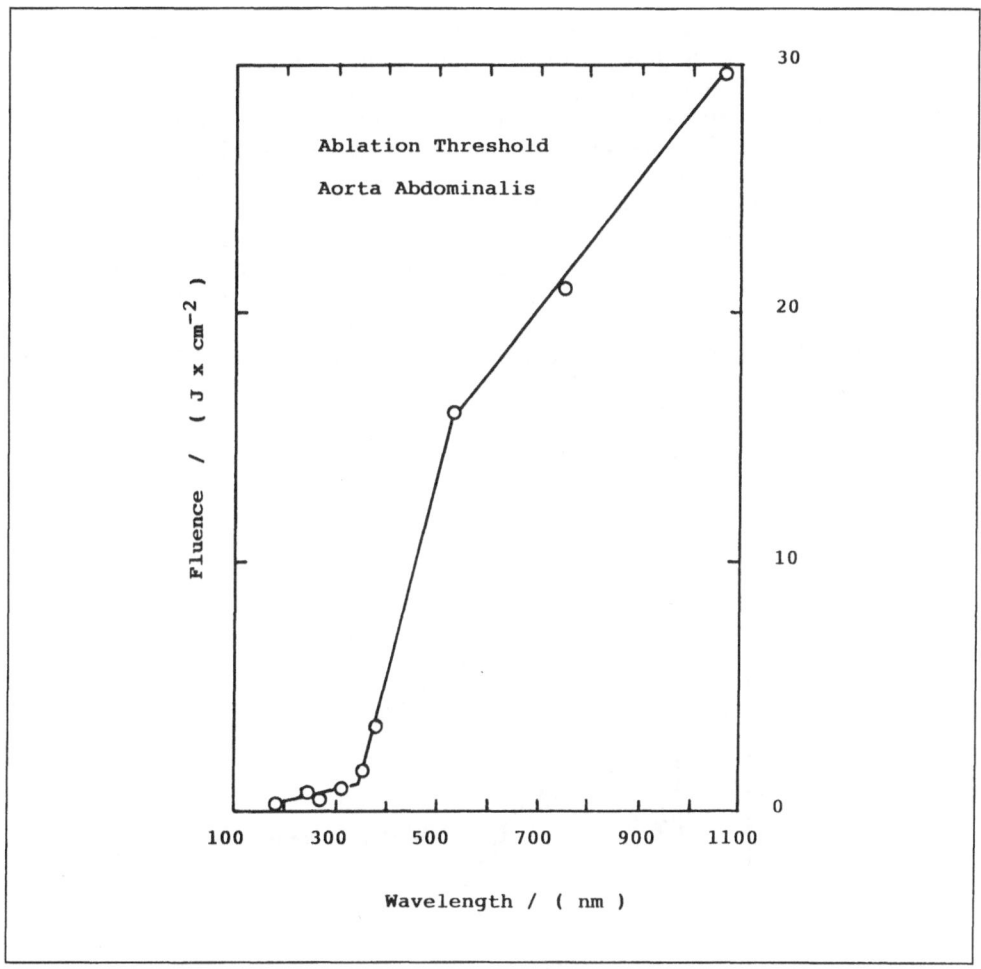

Fig. 7. Ablation threshold of aorta abdominalis vs wavelength.

300 ns. Below 400 nm, fluences of less than 3 J cm^{-2} were sufficient to ablate arterial tissue, whereas more than 20 J cm^{-2} were necessary for wavelengths above 800 nm [25].

Recently, it was shown that about 10 J cm^{-2} were sufficient for tissue removal from the distal aorta with a pulsed Ho:Tm:Cr:YAG laser at 2.13 μm and a pulse duration of 100 to 150 μs (14).

Laser temporal pulse shape

Another important parameter for laser/tissue-interaction is the temporal pulse shape of pulsed laser systems. Liquid or gas lasers normally follow the pulse shapes of their pump-pulse sources, but in solid-state laser systems high- or low-gain laser material can be discriminated that follow, more or less, the temporal shape of their excitation medium. Figure 8 displays this situation for three different laser materials, consisting of Nd:YAG, Er:YAG, and Cr:BeAl$_2$O$_4$ (alexandrite).

The exciting flashlamp pulse with a sketched temporal shape of approx. 500 to 1000 µs duration increases the stored energy in the laser rod until there is sufficient fluorescent radiation bouncing back and forth between the two laser mirrors for laser oscillation to take place (see also Fig. 1). One short pulse of approx. 500–1000 ns duration is released which rapidly reduces the stored energy in a self-quenching process. After a short delay, the stored energy again reaches the threshold condition for oscillation by further absorption of energy from the flashlamp pulse. In this so-called fixed-Q-mode of operation the laser output consists of a series of pulses or spikes, which continue until the pump light can no longer maintain the stored energy at the threshold level.

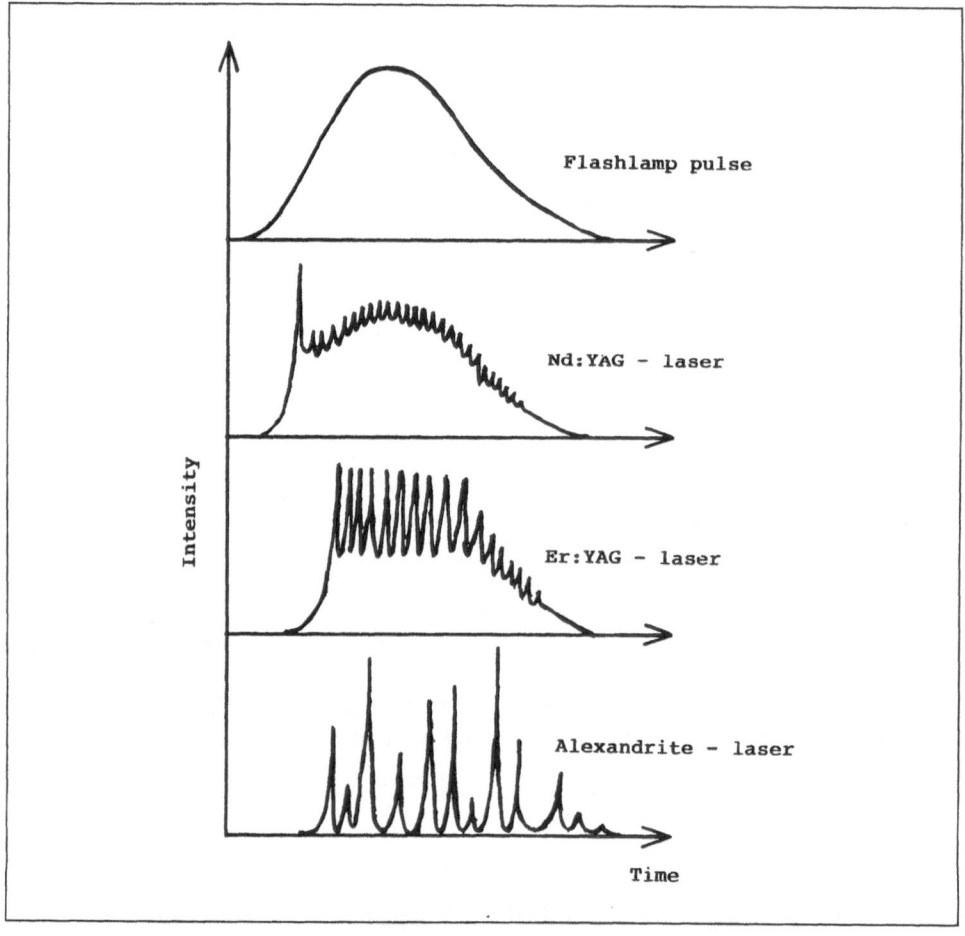

Fig. 8. Temporal pulse shape of different pulsed-laser systems compared to the exciting flashlamp pulse.

For high-gain laser materials, such as Nd:YAG, and high-power pumping rates, spikes are superimposed on the top of a pulse profile which, to a first approximation, follow a form similar to the pumping light pulse. With other laser materials, such as Er:YAG or alexandrite, completely different temporal laser pulse shapes are produced that also depend on the pump power levels used for excitation. Alexandrite, as a low-gain material, shows an extreme statistically varying spiking-behavior, with single pulses of approx. 500 ns duration and very high amplitudes, resulting in extremely high laser peak-power levels. The spikes or relaxation oscillations of this solid-state laser medium produce drilling effects when they interact with tissue material because the total laser pulse energy is subdivided into many single, high-power pulses [20, 30]. These short pulses are mainly responsible for the acoustic transients in laser/tissue-interaction, causing more or less severe acoustomechanical damage to the underlying healthy tissue. Suppressing these spikes by adding optical components like special absorbers or nonlinear materials into the optical resonator can considerably reduce spiking laser oscillations, thus potentially resulting in a more defined ablation process.

Experiments with a spiking Er:YSGG laser at a wavelength of 2.79 μm have shown that the specific energy needed to remove a mass unit of fatty tissue is considerably reduced for a train of single pulses with individual spikes of 500 ns duration, compared to a single pulse with a duration of 100 μs at a constant energy density [2].

Laser beam divergence and radial intensity distribution

Two other laser parameters can also be important for laser/tissue-interaction, especially when the therapeutic laser beam is transmitted via single optical fibers with varying core diameters or via multifiber laser-catheters: the divergence and the radial intensity distribution of the laser beam emitted from the laser resonator. The laser beam, compared to an incoherent light source, is normally regarded as exactly parallel. However, due to the laser resonator configuration and due to the diffraction of the laser beam by apertures, the laser output is divergent to a greater or lesser degree. For that reason, it is not possible to focus a laser beam with an optical lens to a point with no lateral extension.

If the laser is operated in a so-called multi-mode (the normal mode of operation for high-power laser systems) the beam is more divergent than for the so-called single-mode or TEM_{00} operation, where the radial intensity distribution is exactly Gaussian due to apertures within the laser resonator. In this successfully mode-controlled configuration the system has a very low divergence, but also is of low power, and is therefore best suited for fiberoptic coupling to fibers with small core diameters.

Gas lasers, like the CO_2 or the excimer laser, normally have a larger divergence than solid-state lasers like the Nd:YAG laser. Also, their radial intensity distribution looks quite different than that of a solid-state laser. Thus, it is much more difficult for excimer laser radiation to be coupled into small-core-diameter optical fibers with only a simple, single lens, compared to the solid-state laser output which normally has a Gaussian-like shape. Therefore, the coupling efficiency of pulsed or Q-switched solid-state laser radiation to fiberoptic transmitters is much higher than for high-power gas lasers like the excimer laser. In addition, the coupling efficiency is also extremely wavelength- and pulselength-dependent, as can be seen in Figure 9. The data are mainly derived from experiments of Vuman Lasers Ltd. with large-core, multimode, all-silica and plastic-

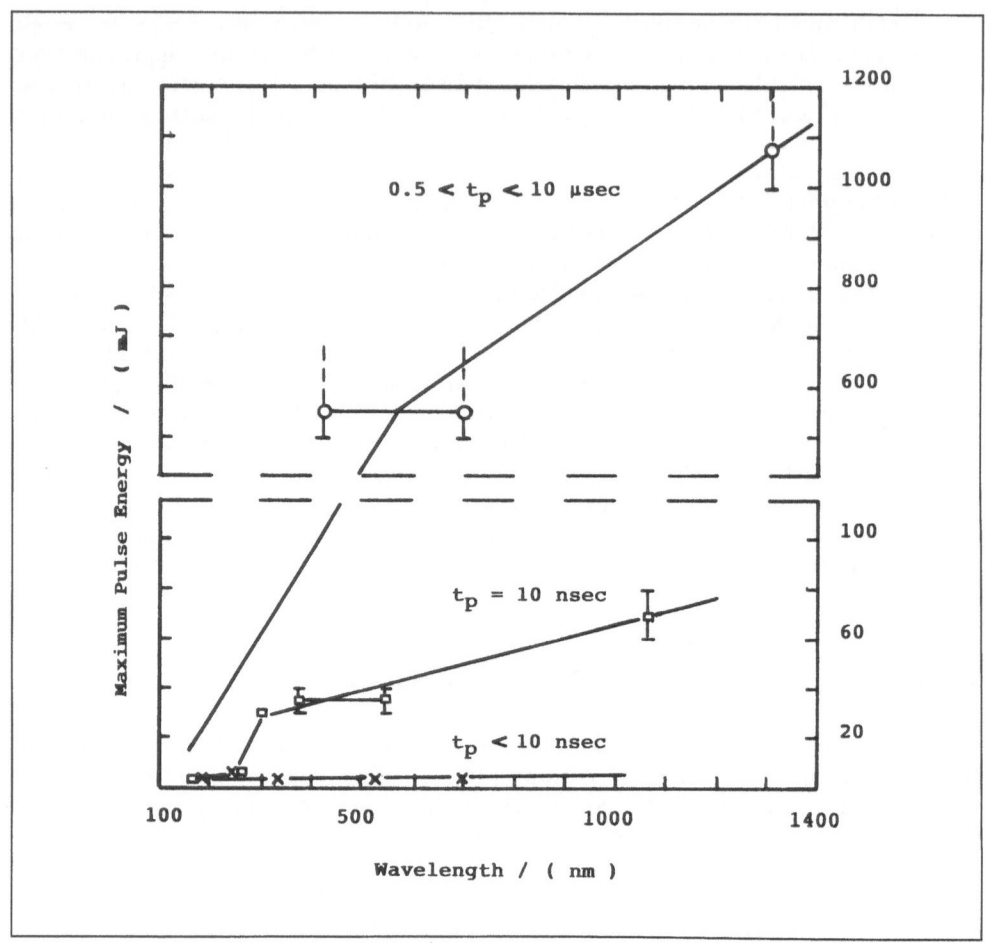

Fig. 9. Maximal transmittable pulse energy of large-core, multimode, all-silica fibers, and plastic-clad, step-index fibers vs wavelength and pulse duration.

clad, step-index fibers, and they give the maximum pulse energy the fiber can transmit without damage (bulk or surface) vs wavelength and pulse duration. For a pulse duration below 10 ns the transmittable pulse energies are quite low (smaller than approx. 10 mJ) and there is nearly no wavelength dependence. This is due to extremely high intensities at the entrance surface of the fiber, which can soon lead to dielectric breakdown and bulk damage. At a pulselength of exactly 10 ns, more pulse energy can be transmitted, especially for longer wavelengths beyond 300 nm. Below that wavelength limit, enhanced fiber absorption of UV light accompanied by fluorescent light emission occurs. In the pulsewidth region of 500 ns to about 10 μs silica fibers are best suited for high-power light transmission, and can transmit pulse energies of more than 1 Joule. Even in the critical UV region below 300 nm the transmittable pulse energy is relatively high [32].

New laser systems for angioplasty

Besides the laser systems already used in angioplastic procedures (with the excimer laser being the most extensively employed in clinical trials) other more complex laser systems, such as metalvapor-, chemical-, CO-, TEA-, or even the free-electron laser, are being investigated for their potential use in laser-angioplasty.

A special group of solid-state lasers will also play an important role, because they are easy to handle, are reliable, and can be constructed as compact units that best fit surgical applications. Table 4 gives a small survey of newly developed solid-state laser materials that emit in a wide range of wave lengths, covering the region of approx. 347 to 2940 nm. Some of these laser crystals are tunable (alexandrite, Ti:sapphire, Cr:GSGG, Cr:fosterite, Cr:YAG), some emit at different individual wavelengths (Nd:YLF, Nd:Cr:Er:GSGG, Er:YAP) and most of them can be Q-switched or frequency-doubled with high efficiency.

With the aid of known data from tests of pulsed lasers in angioplasty, some types will be best-suited for in vitro use and then designated for animal or human trials. However, one should not forget that some of these new materials, like Er:YSGG or Er:YAG, need special beam-delivery systems and laser-catheters that are not in general use today. The well-known and approved all-silica fibers for wavelengths of 300 to approx. 2000 nm

Table 4. Emission wavelengths of solid-state laser materials.

Type of Solid-State Laser	Emission Wavelength (nm)
Ruby	694, 347 (2f)
Alexandrite (t)	720–860, 360–430 (2f)
Ti:Sapphire (t)	700–1100
Cr:GSGG (t)	730–900
Nd:YLF	1047, 1053, 1313, 1321
Nd:Cr:Er:GSGG	1060, 2800, 2830
Nd:Glass	1060, 1370
Nd:Cr:GSGG	1061, 1335
Nd:YAG	1064, 1320, 532 (2f)
Nd:YAP	1079
Cr:Fosterite (t)	1167–1345
Cr:YAG (t)	1350–1450
Er:Glass	1540
Er:YAP	1663, 1677, 1705, 1729 2920, 2730, 2630
Er:YLF	1730
Tm:Cr:YAG	2015
Ho:Tm:Er:YAG	2060
Ho:Tm:Cr:YAG	2080, 2123
Ho:YSGG	2090
Ho:YAG	2120
Er:YSGG	2790
Er:Cr:YSGG	2794
Er:YLF	2800
Er:YAG	2940

(t = tunable; 2f = frequency-doubled)

must be exchanged by mid-infrared fibers like chalcogenide, zirconium fluoride, and thallium or silver halides. These new materials have to prove their applicability in laser-angioplasty with pulsed lasers and high peak powers [1, 15].

An ideal laser for laser-angioplasty?

The question of if there already exists an ideal laser for laser-angioplasty in coronary or peripheral artery disease, when we once more consider the complex relationship of the different laser parameters to tissue ablation, cannot yet be answered.

What we know is that, until now, no data exists to indicate that the quality of laser ablation is largely wavelength-dependent; however, if it is clear that the efficiency of laser ablation varies quantitatively as a function of wavelength. Wavelength, per se, does not appear to be a critical factor in determining the optimal laser for laser-angioplasty. Where wavelength is a critical factor, is the problem of save and efficient fiberoptic transmission of laser radiation, as the laser source itself represents only one of many other components in a complete clinical system. Even the transmission characteristics of individual laser lines in blood do not predict the ability to accomplish laser ablation in a blood field, as it was demonstrated by Isner and co-workers.

On the other hand, a critical feature of an ideal laser system is the way in which laser energy is delivered to the lesion. It is important that thermal injury to the vessel wall be prevented, thus reducing the likelihood of recurrent atheroslerotic stenosis. A improved preservation of structural tissue and fewer thrombogenic residual surfaces can reduce the risk of acute thrombotic occlusion. Vascular spasm, a very frequent consequence of cw-laser irradiation, can only be prevented by pulsed laser radiation. Pulsed lasers with high peak powers can also more effectively ablate heavily calcified lesions. However, the upper limit of the pulse duration that produces ablation without thermal injury is still undefined. Experiments have shown that a pulse duration of up to 1 µs may be used without risk of thermal injury.

Further criteria for an ideal laser in angioplasty should also include compactness and user-friendliness and last, but not least, cost.

References

1. Arai R, Kikuchi M, Mizuno K et al. (1988) Laser angioplasty using carbon monoxide lasers. Optical Fibers in Medicine III, SPIE-906: 282–287
2. Artjushenko VG, Dianov EM, Konov VI et al. (1989) Promising laser fiber systems for surgery. Optical Fibers in Medicine IV, SPIE-1067: 233–241
3. Berlien HP, Biamino G, Dörschel K et al. (1989) Laser angioplasty. Physical and Technical Problems, Biotronic 1: 46–50
4. Bonner RF, Smith PD, Leon M et al. (1986) Quantification of tissue effects due to a pulsed Er:YAG laser at 2.9 µm with beam delivery in a wet field via zirconium fluoride fibers. Optical Fibers in Medicine II, SPIE-713: 2–5
5. Bonner RF, Prevosti LG, Leon MB et al. (1988) New source for laser angioplasty: Er:YAG laser pulses transmitted through zirconium fluoride optical fiber catheters. Optical Fibers in Medicine III, SPIE-906: 288–293

6. Borst C (1987) Percutaneous recanalization of arteries: Status and prospects of laser angioplasty with modified fibre tips. Lasers Med Sci 2: 137–151
7. Choy DSJ, Stertzer SH, Myler RK et al. (1984) Human coronary laser recanalization. Clin Cardiol 7: 377–381
8. Choy DSJ (1988) History of lasers in angioplasty. Advances in Laser Medicine I, First German Symposium on Laser Angioplasty, Biamino G, Müller GJ, 56–64
9. Cross FW, Al-Dhahir RK, Dyer PE et al. (1987) Time-resolved photoacoustic studies of vascular tissue ablation at three laser wavelengths. Appl. Phys. Lett. 50: 1019–1021
10. Cross FW, Al-Dhahir RK, Dyer PE (1988) Ablative and acoustic response of pulsed UV laser-irradiated vascular tissue in a liquid environment. J. Appl. Phys. 64: 2194–2201
11. Esterowitz L, Hoffmann CA, Tran DC et al. (1986) Angioplasty with a laser and fiber optics at 2,94 μm. Optical and Laser Technology in Medicine, SPIE-605: 32–36
12. Gemert van MJC, Welch AJ, Bonnier JJM et al. (1986) Some physical concepts in laser angioplasty. Sem Intervent Radiol 3: 27–38
13. Harnoss BM, Kar H, Müller G et al. (1988) Microspectral photometry of atherosclerotic vessels. Advances in Laser Medicine I, First German Symposium on Laser Angioplasty. In: Biamino G, Müller GJ (Eds) ecomed, pp 157–169
14. Haase KK, Hassenstein S, Steiger E et al. (1991) Holmium laser angioplasty: Evaluation of a new solid state laser for ablation of atherosclerotic plaque. Lasers Surg Med 11: 232–234
15. Haase KK, Steiger E, Duda S et al. (1991) Alexandrite laser-angioplasty: A study on fiber conduction and tissue effects. Lasers Med Sci 6: 183–188
16. Herziger G (1986) Physics of laser materials processing. High Power Lasers and Their Industrial Applications, SPIE-650: 188–194
17. Isner JM, Clarke RH (1984) The current status of lasers in the treatment of cardiovascular disease. IEEE J Quant Electr QE-20: 1406–1420
18. Isner JM, Fields CD, Clarke RH (1988) Cardiovascular laser therapy; The optimal laser. Advances in Laser Medicine I, First German Symposium on Laser Angioplasty, Biamino G, Müller GJ, 65–69
19. Karsch KR, Haase KK, Mauser M et al. (1988) Percutaneous transluminal excimer laser coronary angioplasty. Dtsch. med. Wschr. 114: 1183–1187
20. Koechner W (1976 u. 1988) Solid-State Laser Engineering. Springer Series in Optical Sciences, Vol. 1, Springer Verlag Berlin, Heidelberg, New York
21. Kolbe T, Hibst R, Steiner R (1989) Untersuchungen zu Parametern der Excimer-Laser-Angioplastie in Bezug auf Effizienz und Gewebeschäden. Verhandlungsbericht Deutsche Gesellschaft für Lasermedizin, 36–47
22. Lilge L, Radtke W, Nishioka NS (1989) Pulsed holmium laser ablation of cardiac valves. Lasers Surg Med 9: 458–464
23. Litvack F, Grundfest WS, Goldenberg T et al. (1988) Pulsed laser angioplasty: Wavelength, power and energy dependencies relevant to clinical application. Lasers Surg Med 8: 60–65
24. Murphy-Chutorian D, Kosek J, Mok W et al. (1985) Selective absorption of ultraviolet laser energy by human atherosclerotic plaque treated with tetracycline. Am J Cardiol 55: 1293–1297
25. Müller G, Berlien HP, Biamino G et al. (1988) Photoablation threshold of human aorta as a function of wavelength. LASER-Optoelectronics in Medicine, Waidelich W and R, 38–41
26. Prince MR, Deutsch TF, Mathews-Roth MM et al. (1986) Preferential light absorption in atheromas in vitro: Implications for laser angioplasty. J Clin Invest 78: 295–302
27. Sanborn TA (1988) Current clinical and experimental research using cardiovascular lasers. Lasers Surg Med: News and Advances: 26–35
28. Spears JR (1986) Percutaneous laser treatment of atherosclerosis: An overview of emerging techniques. Cardiovasc Intervent Radiol 9: 308–312
29. Srinivasan R, Leigh WJ (1982) Ablative photodecompositions: action of far-ultraviolet (193 nm) laser radiation on polyethylene terephthalate films. J. Am. Chem. Soc. 104: 6784–6785
30. Steiger E, Kuper JW (1988) A Q-switched alexandrite laser for laser induced shock wave lithotripsy (LISL) – Basics and in vitro studies. Laser Med Surg 2: 43–47
31. Steiger E, Haase KK, Wehrstein M (1989) Comparison of the interaction of free-running and Q-switched Nd:YAG and alexandrite laser radiation with atherosclerotic tissue. Verhandlungsbericht Deutsche Gesellschaft für Lasermedizin, 18–25

32. Taylor RS, Leopold KE, Brimacombe RK et al. (1988) Dependence of the damage and transmission properties of fused silica fibers on the excimer wavelength. Appl. Opt. 27: 3124–3134
33. Weber HP, Lüthy W (1986) 3 µm solid state laser for medical applications. European Conference on Optics, Optical Systems and Applications, SPIE-701: 138–145

Author's address:
Dipl.-Phys. E. Steiger
E. Steiger Lasertechnik GmbH
Spatzenwinkel 7
8038 Gröbenzell, FRG

18

Laser-Tissue Interactions in Laser Angioplasty

J. D. Haller, R. Srinivasan

UVTech Associates, Yorktown Heights, New York, USA

In order to understand the potential, as well as the limitations, in using a laser for angioplasty, it is essential for the physician to have at least a basic understanding of the events that occur as the light energy of the laser is transferred into the biologic tissue within the vessel. That said, it is at once obvious that this·is an enormous subject which encompasses several different dicta which include laser physics, molecular biology, and those branches of clinical medicine that treat cardiovascular disease. Furthermore, our knowledge of the physics involved is incomplete, and there is much that is not known about the biology. Ultimately, the clinical physician can judge his results from simple observation of the complications, recurrences, and failures, without the need to be a physicist. However, in order to avoid needless and futile applications, as well as to reduce patient mortality, it will be helpful if he understands the basic physics and chemistry behind the interaction phenomena. This is also useful to the physician in understanding the marketing claims of different equipment manufacturers. In this chapter, we will describe these physico-chemical factors as they apply to laser angioplasty, and relate them to what is currently known about the initiation of vessel-wall injury and the hyperplastic biologic response that results in restenosis.

In general, the transfer of the light energy into the tissue depends on three factors: the wavelength of the laser radiation, its power density, and the chemical and physical structure of the target. In addition to being interdependent, each of these factors is dependent upon other variables.

The physicist attributes a duality to light energy in that it can be made up of both waves of electro-magnetic radiation and particles of energy with no mass, called photons. Laser photons, which are of practical use in surgery, range in wavelength from the infrared (10.7 μm or 10 700 nm) to the ultraviolet (193 nm). The energies of the photons that are radiated by lasers in use or under clinical investigation are shown in Fig. 1. The wavelength of the laser light is related to the energy of the photon by the formula:

$$E = hc/\lambda, \quad (1)$$

where E is the energy of the photon, h is a universal constant called Planck's constant, and c is the velocity of light. This equation points out the inverse relationship between the energy of a photon and its wavelength. On a per photon basis, infrared lasers are the least energetic, while ultraviolet lasers (which are often simply referred to as "excimer lasers") contain the most energy. This is quantitatively shown in Fig. 1. This inherent energy content of the photon is of great importance in determining its interaction with tissue.

The radiant energy from the laser may come in a continuous stream in which case it is referred to as cw (continuous wave) or it may be intermittent, in which case it is referred to as "pulsed". This aspect of the laser has a profound influence on the power density which influences laser-tissue interactions. The photon may be viewed

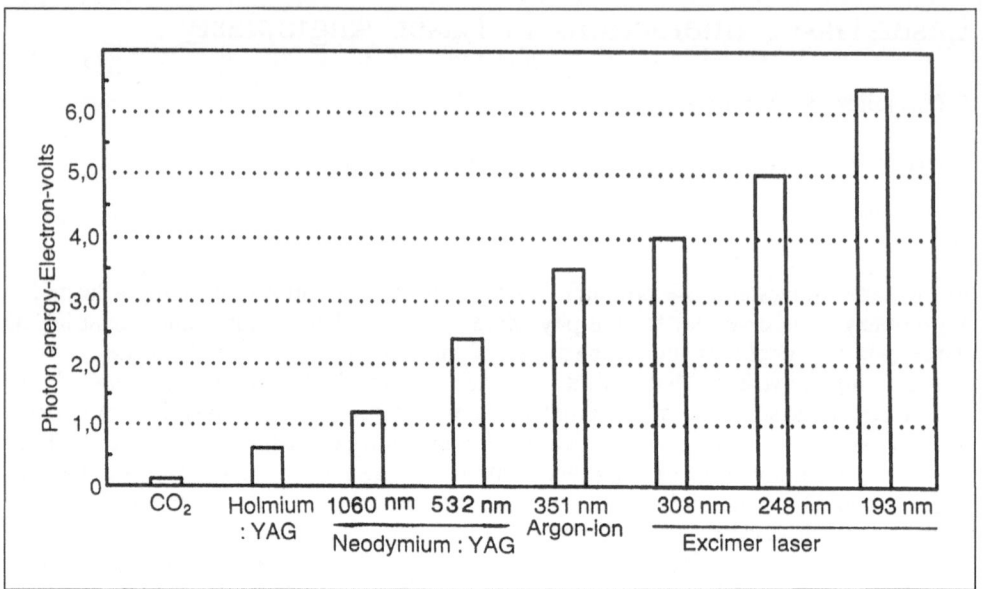

Fig. 1. Energy in electron-volts of photons from lasers currently in use or under investigation for medical applications.

simply as a chemical reagent which interacts with the tissue and alters its chemistry. It then becomes clear that the concentration of the photons which constitutes the "dose" of the reagent strongly affects the rate of the interaction. This concentration is referred to as the *power density*. The power density is expressed in watts per cm^2 of the radiation falling on the tissue site. CW lasers operate in the range from milliwatts to many kilowatts per cm^2 while pulsed lasers, as used in laser angioplasty, operate from 1 to a few hundred million watts/cm^2 (1–100 Megawatts/cm^2) of power density. The importance of the power density level on the nature of the laser-tissue interaction is discussed later in this article.

The transfer of energy or the laser-tissue interactions begins when the laser light strikes the tissue target. The light may be absorbed, reflected, scattered, or transmitted. Usually, all of these processes occur temporally in parallel to varying degrees. Only those photons that are absorbed by the tissue lead to a laser-induced tissue modification. The process of absorption through a medium that does not significantly scatter the light is given by the formula:

$$I_{(transmitted)} = I_{(incident)} \, e^{-\alpha l}, \quad (2)$$

where I is the intensity of the light beam, 1 is the thickness of the tissue through which it passes, and α is a characteristic property of the tissue and is called its absorptivity. When the medium has a strong scattering component, a more complex relationship between the incident intensity and the absorption has to be used [1]. Tissue absorbs light energy in a characteristic fashion which depends upon the chromophores (= absorption centers) that it contains. In addition, water has its own absorption pattern. Since water is the major component of biologic tissue, this factor becomes important in any laser-tissue interaction. The differences in the absorption properties of the tissues of the vessel

20

wall and plaque are minimal, especially at the energy density levels that are needed, although several investigators have attempted to utilize such differences for detection of the atheroma to aim the beam [2, 3, 4]. The fact that the calcium phosphate particles that become dispersed throughout a developing atheroma contain fas less water than the surrounding tissue is important because the energy: tissue interaction of a such a sample is different from that of purely organic components.

The intensity of the absorption of the laser radiation by the tissue at a given wavelength which is the term α in Eq. (2) has an important consequence in the nature of the laser-tissue interaction. If the absorption is strong, the photons penetrate to a depth of only 1/10 th to 1/100 th of a millimeter from the surface of the tissue. This tends to minimize the thermal damage to the underlying areas since the diffusion of heat from the laser photons is kept to a minimum. For the same reason, shortening the pulse also tends to minimize the thermal damage in the lateral direction, i. e., along the surface in the areas that adjoin the exposed area.

The wavelengths of infrared photons correspond in energy to vibrational and rotational excitation of the molecules of the target tissue. Such energy, which in common language is referred to as "heat", is rapidly redistributed among the molecules and raises the temperature of the tissue. At power densities of a kilowatt/cm^2 or more, especially when the exposure time is in milliseconds or longer, the temperature of the exposed region can rise to well above the boiling point of water on the same time scale. Here the primary absorber of the photon becomes an important consideration. Short-pulsed solid state lasers in the near-infrared range, such as the Er: YAG and the Ho: YAG, are well-suited in wavelength to be absorbed selectively by the water component in tissue. The output of the CO_2 laser is also in the infrared range at a wavelength that is strongly absorbed by water, but the lack of a suitable means to deliver this energy inside the blood vessel has eliminated its application in laser angioplasty.

When photons from ultraviolet lasers (which are mainly the excimer lasers) are used, the nature of the absorption process becomes fundamentally different. It leads to excitation of the electrons that hold the atoms of the structural molecules together. This is called *electronic excitation* for obvious reasons. It conveys the energy of the photon directly to the bonding electrons and facilitates the break-up of these bonds. The process of excitation itself can cause the bond-break or it can happen subsequently in a few billionths of a second. A whole field of study called *photochemistry* has grown over the past century, because chemical changes that are brought about by ultraviolet photons are pervasive in our life; they include beneficial effects such as photosynthesis and sun-tanning, as well as deleterious effects such as air pollution (photochemical "smog") and destruction of the ozone layer in the stratosphere. It must be pointed out that while electronic excitation is due to a specific excitation process at a given wavelength, the reactions that follow need not be equally specific. Heating effects during ultraviolet excitation are entirely common. This may be either due to inefficiencies in the bond-breaking process so that photons that fail to break a bond merely heat the molecule, or the bond energy is considerably less than the energy of the photon so that the excess is available for heating.

The laser-tissue interaction is a collective process in which a stream of photons interacts with a section of tissue. The density of the photon stream which is the power density that was already mentioned, is one of the two factors that control the density of excited molecules in the tissue at the instant the light beam strikes the tissue. At the power levels at which lasers operate, the laser-tissue interaction is by no means limited to a given molecule being excited by just one photon, but two- and even multi-

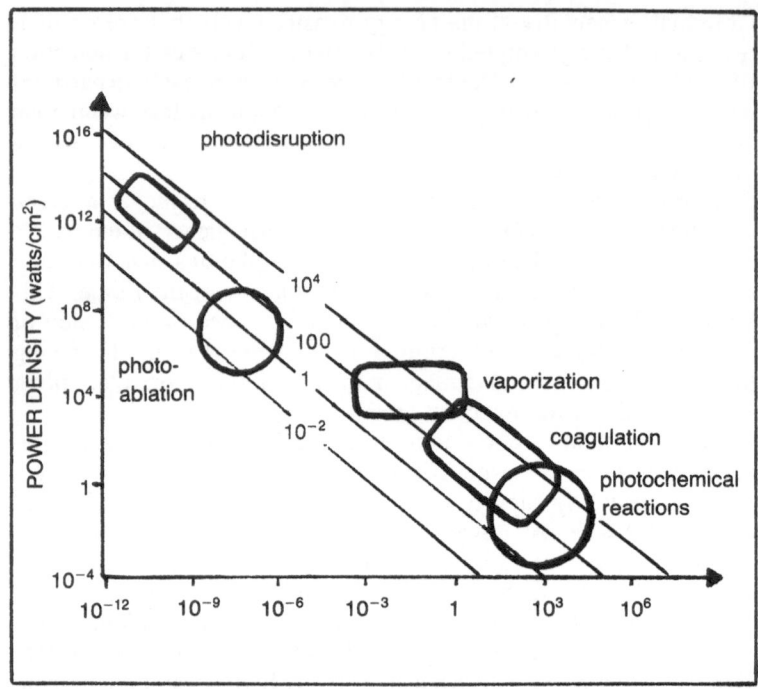

Fig. 2. A matrix showing how different laser-tissue interactions relate to the power densities and pulse widths of the laser. Both scales are logarithmic. The diagonal lines connect points of constant energy density (fluence) in joules/cm^2.

photon excitations become possible. This is the significance of the power density in understanding the chemistry that is brought about by the laser. Figure 2 is a plot of matrix of power densities and pulse widths that are currently being employed in the gamut of laser-tissue interactions. In order to understand this figure, it should be kept in mind that:

$$\text{Fluence} = \text{Energy deposited/area}, \quad (3)$$

where the energy deposited is usually expressed in Joules (4.2 Joules = 1 calorie). Again:

$$\text{Power density} = \text{Energy deposited/area} \times \text{time}, \quad (4)$$

so that:

$$\text{Power density} = \text{Fluence/time}. \quad (5).$$

The shorter the time (i. e., pulse width) in which a given amount of energy (fluence) is delivered to the tissue, the more likely it will lead to excitation of a molecule by more than one photon. Ablative photodecomposition and photodisruption depend strongly on such multi-photon processes. The same amount of energy, if delivered in a longer pulse, (towards the right of the figure) results in simple, one-photon reactions and heating effects. In all this discussion, the wavelength of the photon should always be kept in mind for reasons which have already been explained.

In the clinical application of coronary laser angioplasty, at present are only two basic interactions between the photon beam and the arterial wall (including the atheroma) that have to be considered. These are the interactions that are brought about by a pulsed, infrared laser whose photons are absorbed predominantly by the water in the tissue, and by a pulsed, ultraviolet laser whose photons are absorbed exclusively by the organic bodies. Other modes of laser-tissue interactions have been attempted in laser angioplasty, and they are mentioned here for their historical interest. The earliest attempts were made with a cw argon ion laser which emitted radiation in the visible spectrum. Extensive use was also made of a fiber-optic device in which the end of the fiber was capped by metal so that the beam did not really interact directly with the tissue, but merely served to heat the metal tip for short periods of time; this is not a laser-tissue interaction. More recently, in a modification of this procedure, the laser beam both heated the tip and escaped partially to interact with the tissue. Here again, the output of the laser was in the visible spectrum so that the interaction of the photons with the tissue was probably thermal in nature.

Before discussing the two laser-tissue interaction modes that are currently available in commercial instruments for laser angioplasty, it is relevant to examine the pathology of the atherosclerotic lesion that obstructs the coronary artery and has been selected for laser treatment [5]. The normal coronary artery consists, from its inner lumen outwards, of an endothelial layer, a basal lamina, and then an internal elastic lamella that by definition demarcates the boundary between the media. This layer contains smooth muscle cells, elastin, and collagen, and is bounded on its outer limits by the external elastic lamella which separates this layer from the outer adventitia. This outermost layer consists of fibrocellular connective tissue and is the entry layer for the vessel wall's own nutrient vasa vasora. While the media and adventitia vary considerably in thickness and relative composition of elastin, collagen, and muscle fibers in different locations in the body, all of these constituents are basically chemically similar so far as the laser action is concerned. At the power densities that are needed to ablate plaque within the vascular system, the differences between collagen, muscle cells, and elastin are quite minor. For all practical purposes, they are all organic molecules with a very high water content, and they react to nearly the same laser energy. Normal vessel wall may therefore be considered to be homogenous to laser energy transfer. Blood in between the laser delivery system and various absorption centers (chromophores) within the vessel wall or plaque may influence the amount of energy that is available for absorption. But these situations are really special circumstances that do not alter the basic energy transfer.

Atherosclerotic plaque is altogether a different situation. As it accumulates beneath the intima it is, at first, entirely organic, consisting only of fatty organic molecules in the form of cholesterol. Later, it accumulates more organic material in the form of fibrous tissue and smooth muscle cells. At this stage in the development of the atheroma it is entirely organic and, therefore, homogenous. It reacts to laser energy in a manner that is similar to that of the normal vessel wall. The nature of the absorption process in tissue (in general) for ultraviolet photons and the subsequent chemistry of the interaction have been shown to be quite related to the interaction of these laser photons with synthetic organic polymers [6]. This knowledge has provided a basis for the details of the laser-reaction modes that are described below.

The overall process of using the photon energy of a pulsed laser to cause a transformation in a tissue can be sorted into three individual steps (Fig. 3). These are a) absorption of the photon, b) bond breaking, c) ablation of the products. The last step does not

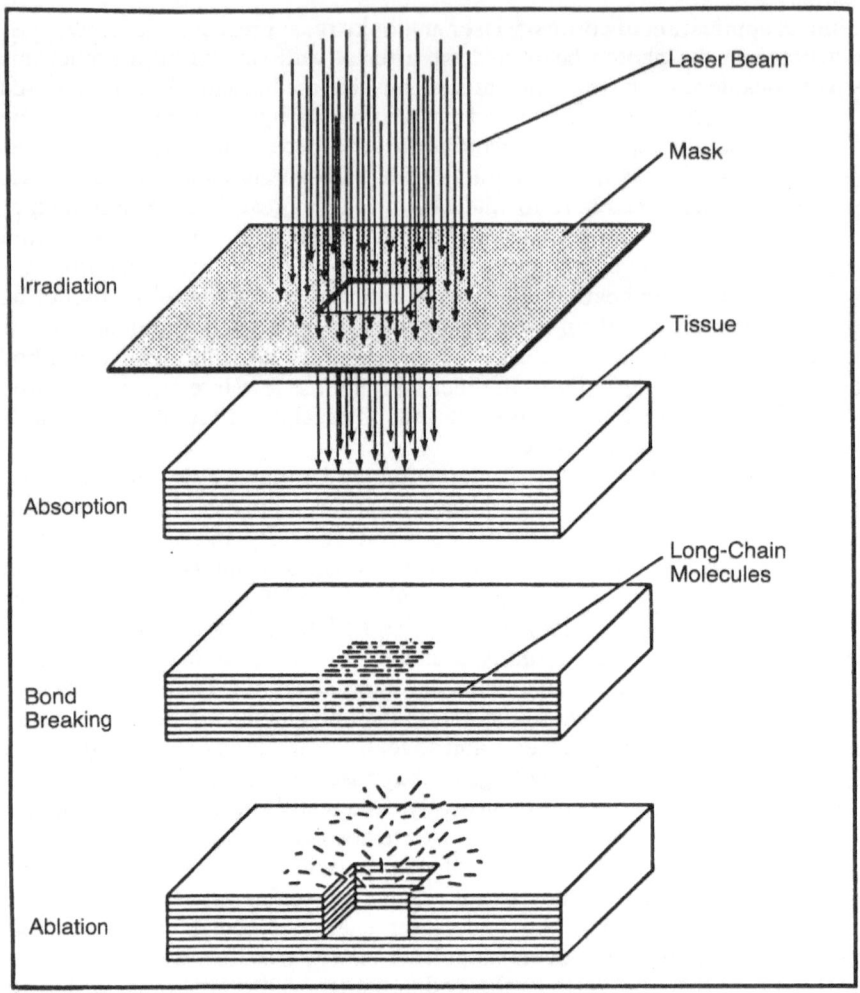

Fig. 3. Hypothetical steps in the interaction of a laser beam with tissue. Top: the laser radiation, which is defined by a mask, is absorbed; Middle: chemical bonds are broken in the tissue by the photon energy; Bottom: the products ablate at supersonic velocities, leaving an etched sample.

always follow, as the first two steps can leave a transformed material in place. Ablation is a miniature explosion that is brought about in the tissue by the sudden build-up of pressure. In turn, this pressure rise, which can momentarily reach 1 000 atm, is caused by three factors: the replacement of the polymorphic structural protein by its decomposition products, which will be a mixture of gases, small molecules, and fragments of the solid protein; an increase in pressure that is due to the vaporization of water if the temperature rises well above the boiling point of water; and a general rise in temperature which is due to the photon energy being converted, in part, to thermal energy. These three factors can work independently and assume different degrees of importance when lasers of different wavelengths are used. This is illustrated in Fig. 4. Ultraviolet radia-

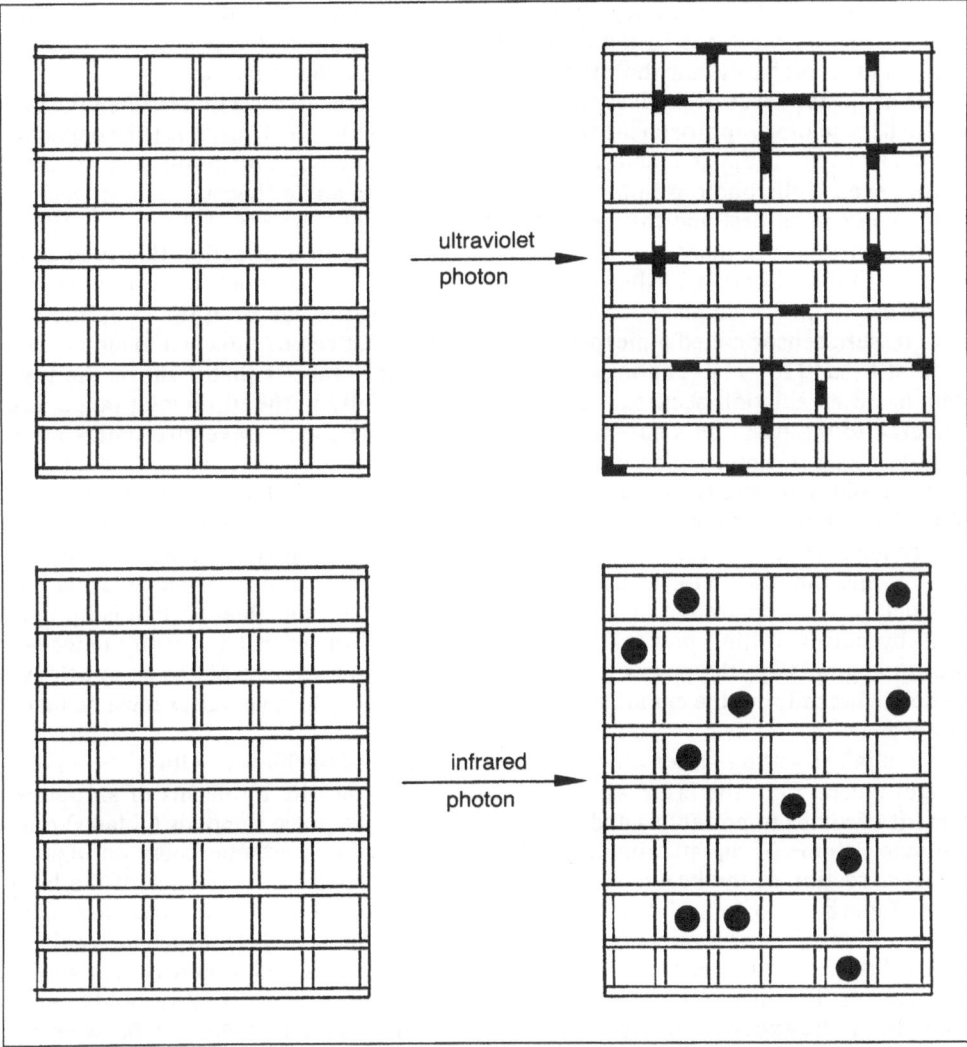

Fig. 4. A comparison of the interaction of ultraviolet photons with tissue (top) with the interaction of infrared photons with tissue (bottom). The mesh represents filaments of structural protein molecules interspersed with the water which constitutes the major part of tissue. When the photons are of ultraviolet wavelengths, absorption is exclusively by the protein, which then undergoes bond-breaking and ablation. The water is expelled mostly in a liquid state, along with the pieces of the protein and its gaseous products. When the photons are of infrared wavelengths, it is the water that absorbs strongly to produce steam. The resulting explosion tears the protein filaments apart.

tion targets the organic material and, therefore, the fragmentation of the protein will be more important than the vaporization of water as the propulsive force. The identification of this mechanism as a photochemical ablation or *ablative photodecomposition* was first described with reference to tissue in 1983 [8]. In the ablation of the cornea by pulsed 193 nm laser radiation this has actually been demonstrated [9]. When the laser wavelength is in the infrared range, it is the water in the tissue that mainly absorbs the radiation and boils; the integrity of the tissue is destroyed as the protein structure is unravelled by the force of the explosion. Local heating of the tissue is a constant factor, but is probably not the primary one in causing the ablation.

The explosive force of the laser ablation is contained in all directions except the one in which the photons approach the surface of the tissue (Fig. 3). Thus, it is to be expected that the force of the ejected material is exactly perpendicular to the tissue surface. This is true, even if the photons approach the surface at an angle, because the process of absorption comes first and this is confined to the surface layers of the tissue. When ablation does occur, there is a shock-wave that travels in a direction that is exactly opposite to the direction of the expelled products, i. e., the shock wave travels into the tissue. Its presence has been detected and its passage has been timed by the use of a pressure sensor called a piezo-electric detector that can be attached to an isolated piece of tissue [10, 11]. The importance of the shock wave is that it shows the time scale in which ablation occurs. If the photons, especially in the ultraviolet range, are delivered to the tissue in a sub-microsecond pulse, the shock wave also builds up in a similar scale of time, which demonstrates that the process of break-up of the tissue is quite rapid. An equally important point of much concern that derives from the study of these shock waves is the potential for shock-induced damage to the artery wall. The shorter the laser pulse, the higher the power density (for a given energy content, see Fig. 2), and the more violent the force of the ablation becomes. Since ablation and its shock wave are paired in magnitude by a physical law, the ablation that is brought about by pulses of high power density cause shock damage that is readily detected. In laser angioplasty, the power densities are kept as low as possible so as to achieve the desired result, but the cumulative action of numerous ablative pulses must be taken into account.

In a clinical setting, laser ablation of the atheroma is achieved with a succession of light pulses from the laser which are delivered to the site by means of an optical fiber. It becomes important to understand that the single pulse removes (ablates) only a minute volume of the atheroma, the cross-section of this volume being defined by the cross-section of the beam, and the depth being related to the fluence of the laser pulse. Figure 5 shows a plot of the depth of the material that is removed per pulse at two different laser wavelength and over a range of fluences [12]. Since the healthy, normal arterial wall is also susceptible to these pulses, its etch-depth is also shown as a function of fluence. A number of points should be noted. There is a threshold fluence which has to be exceeded before there is any ablation. This threshold is the same for the normal vessel wall and the atheroma, but when the magnitude of the fluence rises above the threshold, the two samples show significantly different susceptibility to ablation. The wavelenghts of the photons make an enormous difference, but, in a clinical situation, the optimum wavelength is not neccesarily the one that produces the most ablation, because the delivery of the photon energy to the inside of the artery involves many practical problems which are also a function of the wavelength. At 351 nm, which is one of the wavelengths at which clinical tests of laser angioplasty are presently being carried out, it should be observed (Fig. 5) that the normal wall would be etched to 50% of the depth to which the atheroma would be etched at the same fluence. This shows the serious need to monitor the nature of the target that the tip of the fiber is facing in order to avoid perforations that can be caused by ablation of a healthy portion of the vessel wall.

The exact nature of the process of ablation has been revealed by a photographic technique [13]. The set-up is shown schematically in Figs. 6 and 7. In these experiments,

26

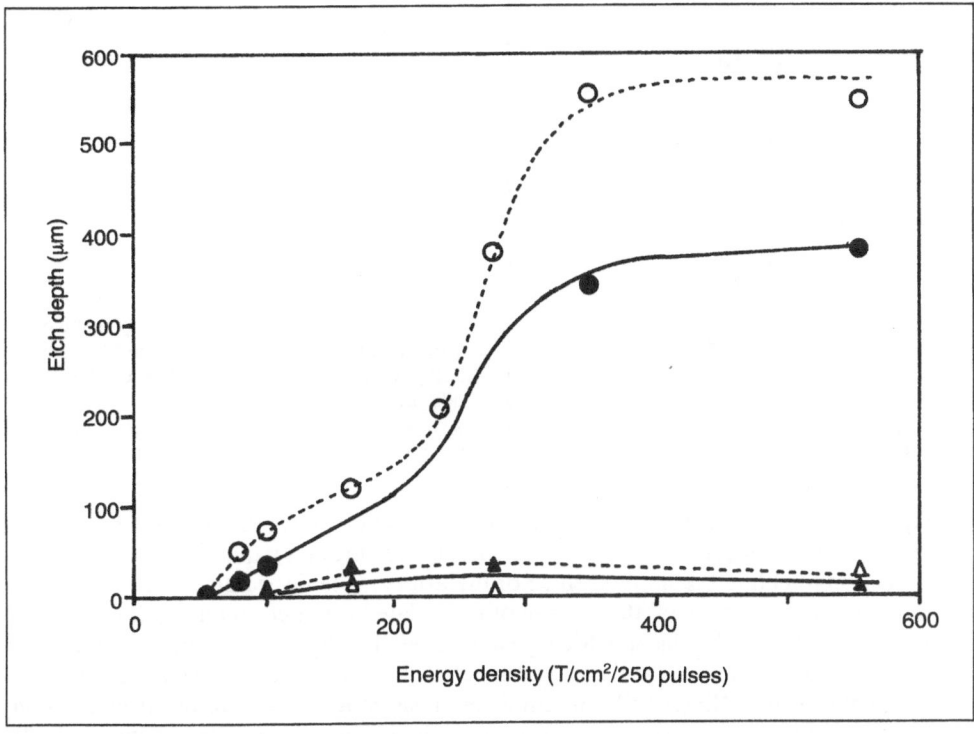

Fig. 5. Etch-curve for normal (continous line) and atheromatous (dashed line) aortic wall at 249 nm and 351 nm. The energy density is the total value for a train of 250 pulses. (Data from [11]).

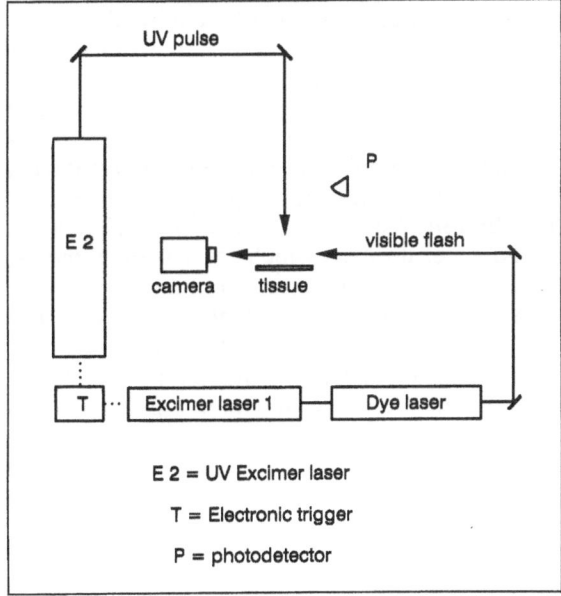

E 2 = UV Excimer laser

T = Electronic trigger

P = photodetector

Fig. 6. Schematic view of set-up for photographing the ablation of tissue. The ablating pulses come from the excimer laser marked E2. The other excimer laser is for "pumping" the dye laser, that is the photographic light source. (A detailed view of the beam delivery is shown in Fig. 7.)

27

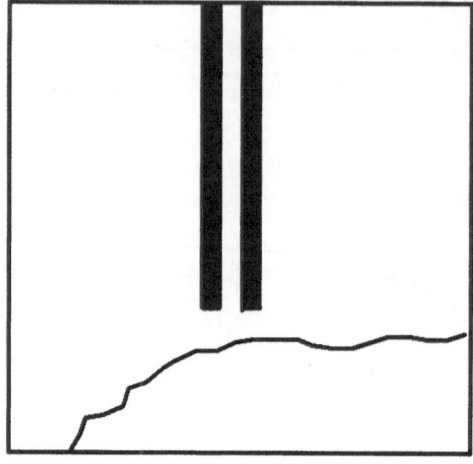

Fig. 7. Schematic view of the delivery of the beam through an optical fiber in the set-up for fast photography of ablation (shown in Fig. 6). The vertically oriented optical fiber is 600-μm thick. Its end, as shown, is 0.5 mm from the surface of the tissue (the area at the bottom of the figure).

which were carried out in vitro from a sample of artery wall that had been removed postmortem, laser energy of 308 nm was channelled through a quartz fiber of 600 μm cross-section to ablate the inner surface of the artery. The laser pulse had a half-width of 30 ns. In order to "freeze" the motion of the ablated products at any time t following the ablation pulse, a dye laser which produced visible light pulses of less than 1 ns duration was used. A timer (trigger) connected to both lasers allowed the dye laser (which provided the "flash" illumination for flash photography) to be fired at a controlled delay after the ultraviolet laser pulse had been fired. The event could be photographed by the light of the dye laser using an ordinary camera which was set up as shown in Fig. 6.

The purpose of these photos was to investigate how ablation occurred when the optical fiber was placed well above the tissue surface, as opposed to when it was in contact with it (Fig. 7). A comparison was also made between ablation of the normal wall and a soft atheroma. Figures 8–11 show these results. Since ablation is an explosion that is brought about by the generation of an enormous pressure inside the tissue, one can expect the products to emerge from the surface at a speed higher than the velocity of sound in air. When this stream meets the air at atmospheric pressure, a blast wave is created which becomes visible because of the great difference in the refractive indices within and outside the gas bubble. This is usually followed, at times of the order of microseconds, by a stream of debris (usually referred to as a "plume") which consists of solid particles of tissue or atheroma and water droplets which are driven by the gas stream. Both the blast wave and the plume slow down as they cool and expand.

Figures 8 and 9 show the effect of pulses of laser light at a constant fluence on normal arterial wall and soft plaque. The blast wave is seen to emerge from the surface in Fig. 8c and expands progressively in the subsequent frames (Figs. 8d–f). Its average velocity is 7.5×10^5 cm/s which is in the supersonic range. In frame Fig. 8b the profile of the blast wave is complex and actually shows an inverted pattern. It is possible that the presence of the fiber, which is only 0.5 mm from the tissue surface, causes a reflection of the blast wave from the fiber end. In frame Fig. 8c, the plume is visible because of its opacity. Its progress in **d**, **e**, and **f** is not clearly outlined, but it is possible to calculate a velocity for only the front edge. This value is 4×10^4 cm/s which is slightly greater than the velocity of sound in air.

In a series of frames in Fig. 9, the ablation of the soft plaque is seen to be much different from the ablation of the artery wall. The blast wave is only faintly seen. The plume emerges in Fig. 9a with a velocity that is similar to that noted in the artery wall, but its density (opacity) is far greater, which suggests that the amount of solid and liquid material that is ablated is also greater. Material is ejected from the surface for as long as 15 μs and the ejected material is seen as a dark "cloud" even at 30 μs.

In Fig. 10, the effect of close contact between the fiber end and the intimal wall is pictured. The blast wave, as it is propelled by rapidly expanding gases at high pressure, manages to escape from the confinement of the fiber and (Figs. 10b–f). In polymer ablation, it has been estimated that the gas pressure that is built up during ablation may be of the order of 100 to 1 000 atm. It is not surprising that gases at such high pressure would escape into the interstices between the fiber and the tissue surface. However, the plume is totally suppressed, and just a trace of debris is visible in Fig. 10d.

Figure 11 shows that when the fiber tip is gently pressed against the surface of the soft plaque, the result is different from that seen in the intimal wall; frames 11 b–e show that there is a violent upheaval of the surface around the fiber tip as the confined gases burst out of the limited volume in which they are formed. The softness of the plaque is undoubtedly an important factor.

In a clinical application of laser pulses for angioplasty, the fiber tip is steadily advanced into the plaque in order to open a channel. To see how the progress of the tip into the plaque affects the ablation that is caused by successive pulses, a series of photos was taken at a constant time delay of 60 μs between the ultraviolet pulse and the "flash" pulse. These results are shown in Fig. 12. The first pulse was fired with the fiber end in contact with the surface of the plaque. As observed in the earlier series (Fig. 11c, d) a violent bursting of the surface is observed. For a second pulse, the fiber tip was *not* advanced. A similar outburst was not seen in this instance (Fig. 12b). Pulse 3 was fired after the fiber tip was advanced until contact with the tissue surface was felt. At this point the fiber end is buried inside the plaque. The ablation is, once again, as violent (Fig. 12c) as with the first pulse. For pulse 4, the fiber tip was not advanced and the ablation process was not violent (Fig. 12d). This series of photographs poses an important problem in the clinical practice of laser angioplasty. The interventional physician who positions the distal end of the laser catheter against a partial or total obstruction in a vessel uses the tactile response that results from firm contact between the fiber and the surface of the tissue as a guide. But as the catheter moves into the material that is being ablated, a tight channel will be formed, which was pointed out by Kar and Biamino [14]. Figure 13 illustrates the problem as set forth by them. The enclosure of the distal end of the catheter into the plaque traps the expanding gases until only a violent ablation can permit their escape. This can cause an unacceptable stress to the walls of the vascular system. As the power of the laser is increased in instances in which the plaque has a certain degree of calcification, the risk to the artery wall can be made worse. Laser guidance systems which offer some method of informing the operator of the pressures that are being encountered at the distal and of the catheter could be beneficial in reducing tissue injury. Although Figs. 7–12 were obtained using an ultraviolet laser, these observations can be equally applicable to any laser source that treats stenosis and occlusions by ablative phenomena. The pressure build-up that precedes ablation may be due to different kinds of laser-tissue interactions, but the effects of ablation depend only on the explosive power behind the phenomenon.

There is no satisfactory model of human atherosclerosis. Animal models produce only cholesterolomas with minimal, if any, inorganic salts. Most studies have therefore

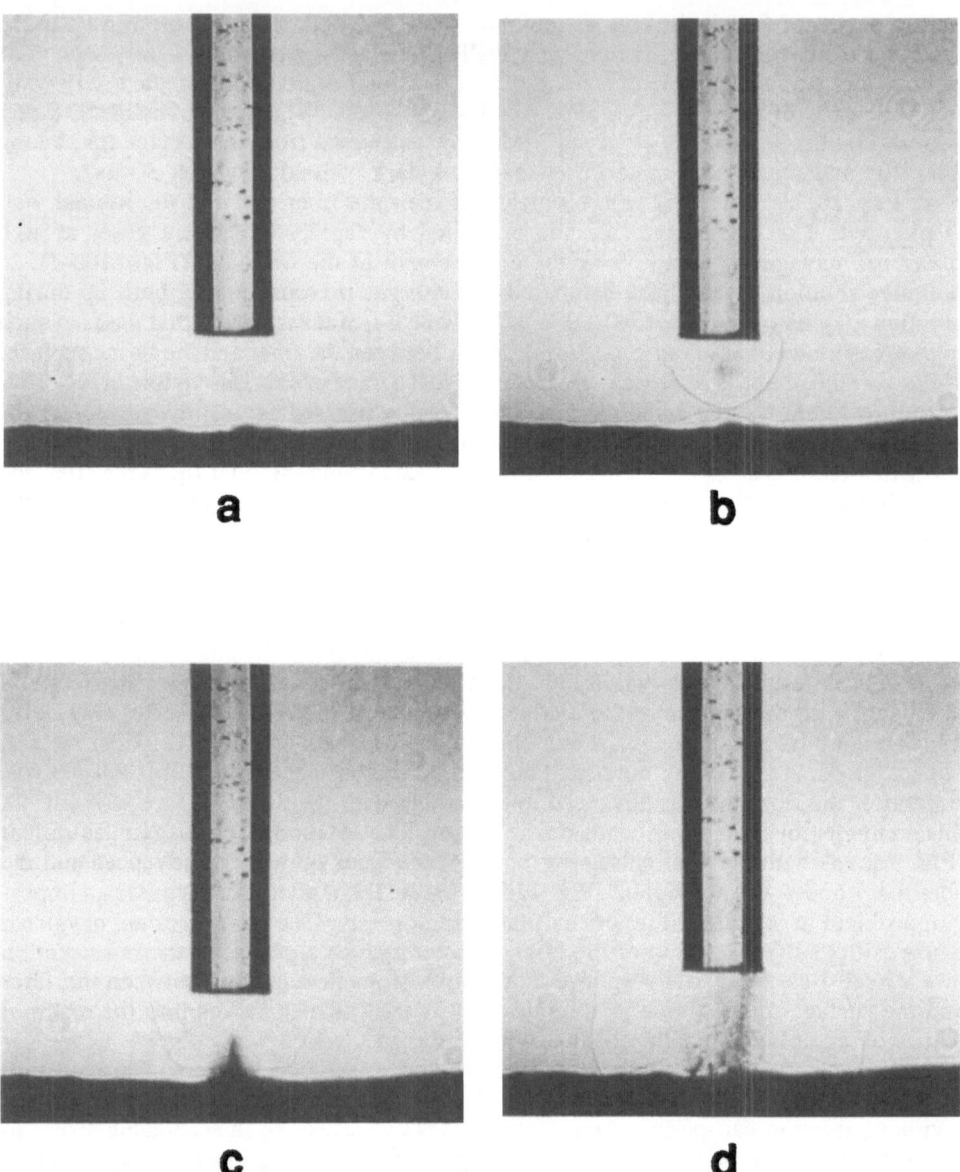

Fig. 8. Ablation of intimal wall by a single UV (308 nm) pulse seen in profile. The frame approximately covers 3 mm × 3 mm. The times represent the delay between the excimer pulse and the dye laser pulse: a) 0 nanosecond, b) 400 ns, c) 750 ns, d) 1 500 μs, e) 3 μs, f) 6 μs, and g) 12 μs.

been done on homogenous animal cholesterol plaques or on strips of human vessels that contain relatively early sub-intimal fatty streaks. Once the severely diseased human vessels are removed at autopsy or at surgery, they are no longer living and a valid biological response cannot be noted. Most studies of the complex lesions of atherosclerosis that cause symptoms have been acute, and performed on dead tissue, such as the photographic series described above. While this type of study gives much

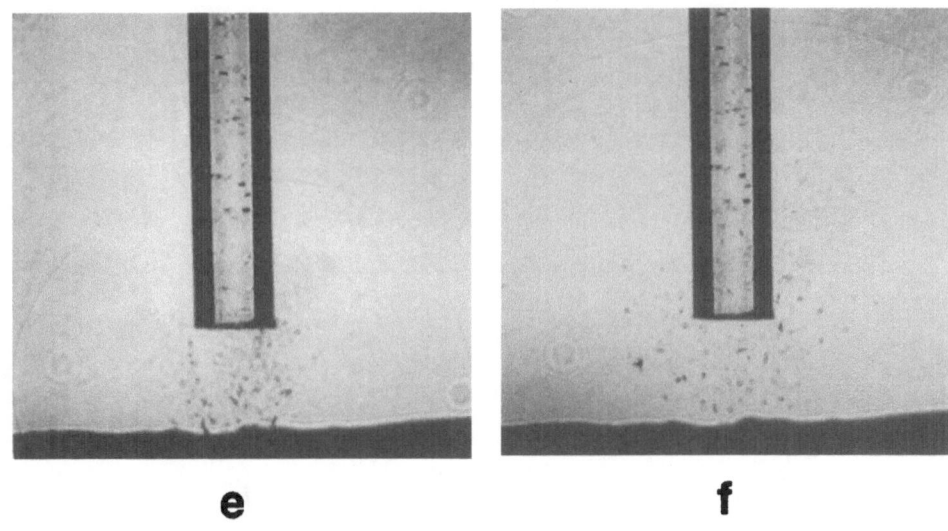

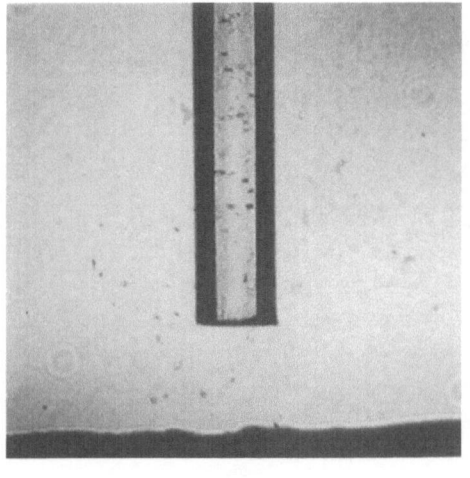

Fig. 8.

valuable information, it is limited, and give only some indication of late biological reactions. In addition. it is apparent by its very nature that the laser destroys the target tissue. So theoretically, for heterogenous targets, it is not possible to know exactly what the target was since it was destroyed. Ultimately, the results of the laser-tissue interaction to remove atherosclerotic plaque have become apparent from the clinical outcome. Although plaque is initially simply a deposition of cholesterol, it evolves

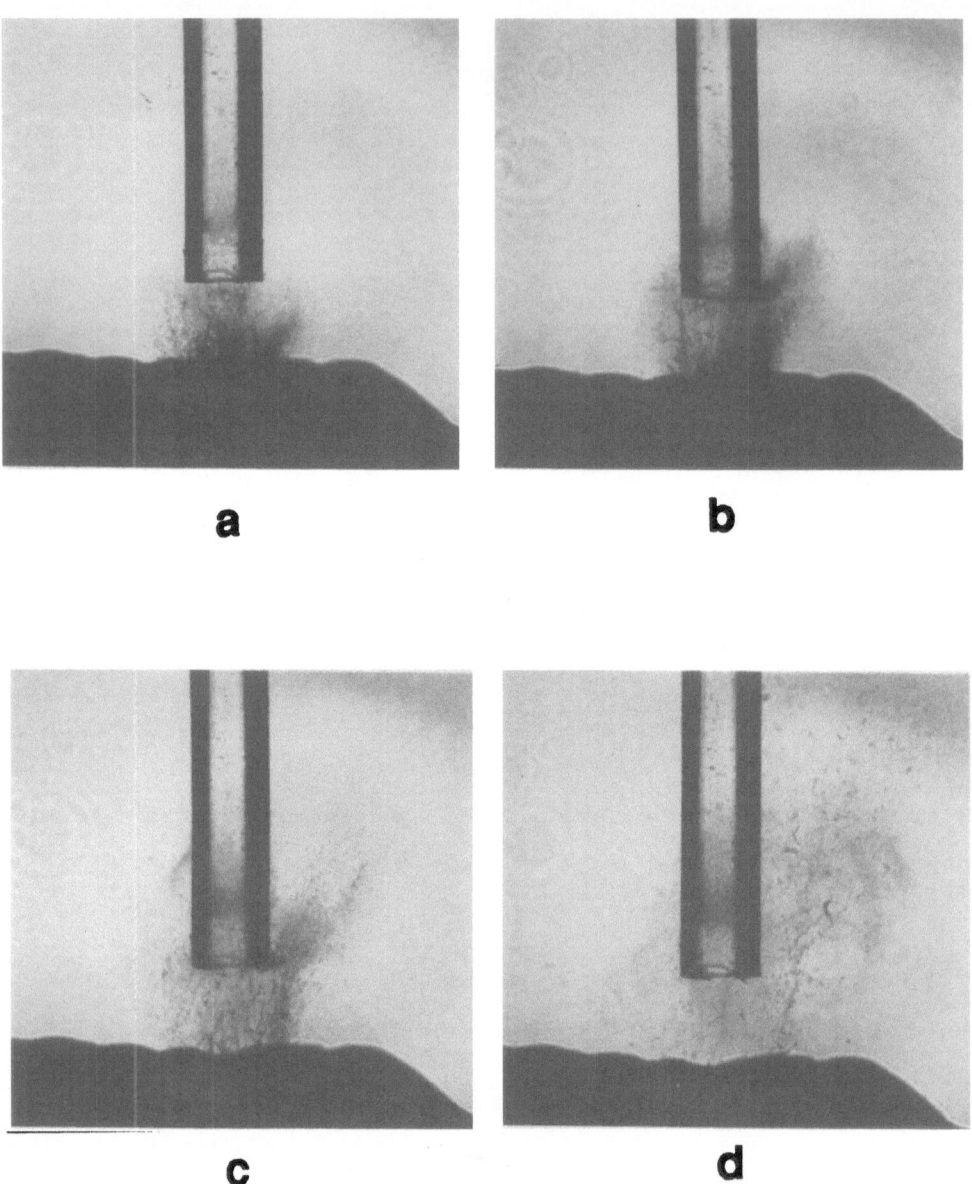

Fig. 9. Ablation of soft plaque by a single UV (308 nm) pulse seen in profile. Magnification as in Fig. 8. The delay times are: a) 1 µs, b) 3 µs, c) 6 µs, d) 15 µs, e) 30 µs, f) 100 µs, and g) ∞ time.

through complex and as yet incompletely understood mechanisms into a complex substance that inevitably contains inorganic calcium salts. Diminution of arterial flow and therefore the onset of symptoms does not occur until the cross-sectional area of the vessel is occluded beyond 75%. The more severe the obstruction, the more symptomatic it becomes and the greater the likelihood that the lesion may contain calcium salts. The presence of the inorganic material is important since the target becomes

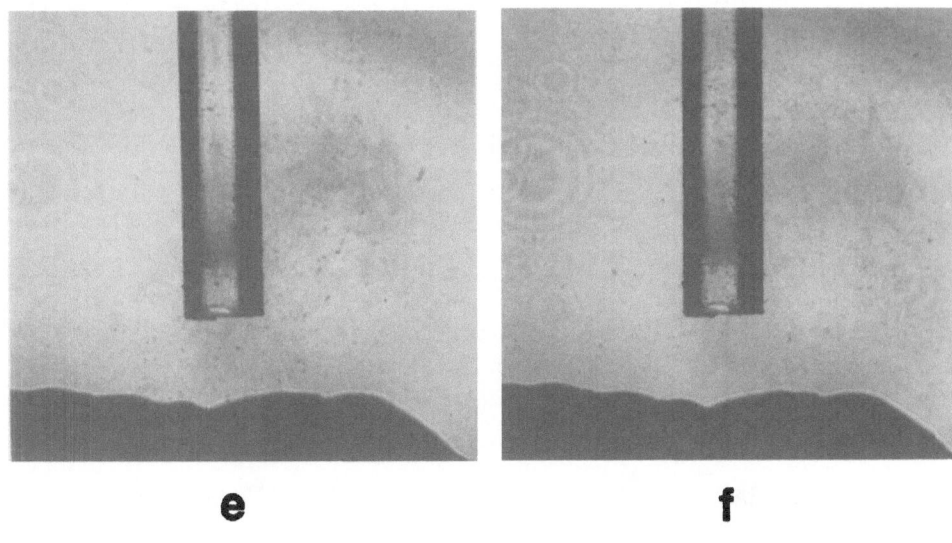

e   f

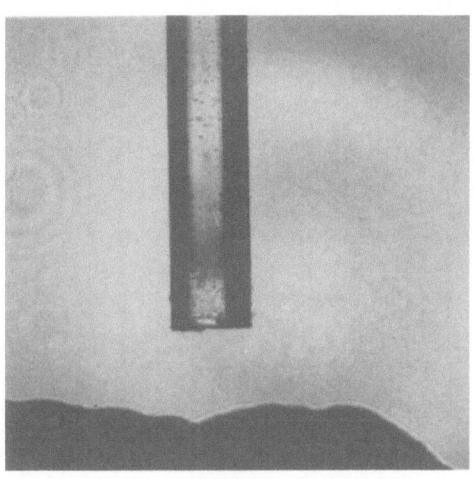

g

Fig. 9.

heterogenous and the relatively simple means of organic tissue ablation no longer applies. In previous studies [15–17], it was reported that when excimer laser energy at short pulse duration, but above the threshold for ablation, strikes pure organic plaque, i. e., fatty streaks, or early cholesterolomas without any inorganic calcium, the reaction is basically non-thermal and is believed to be photochemical. The effect on completely

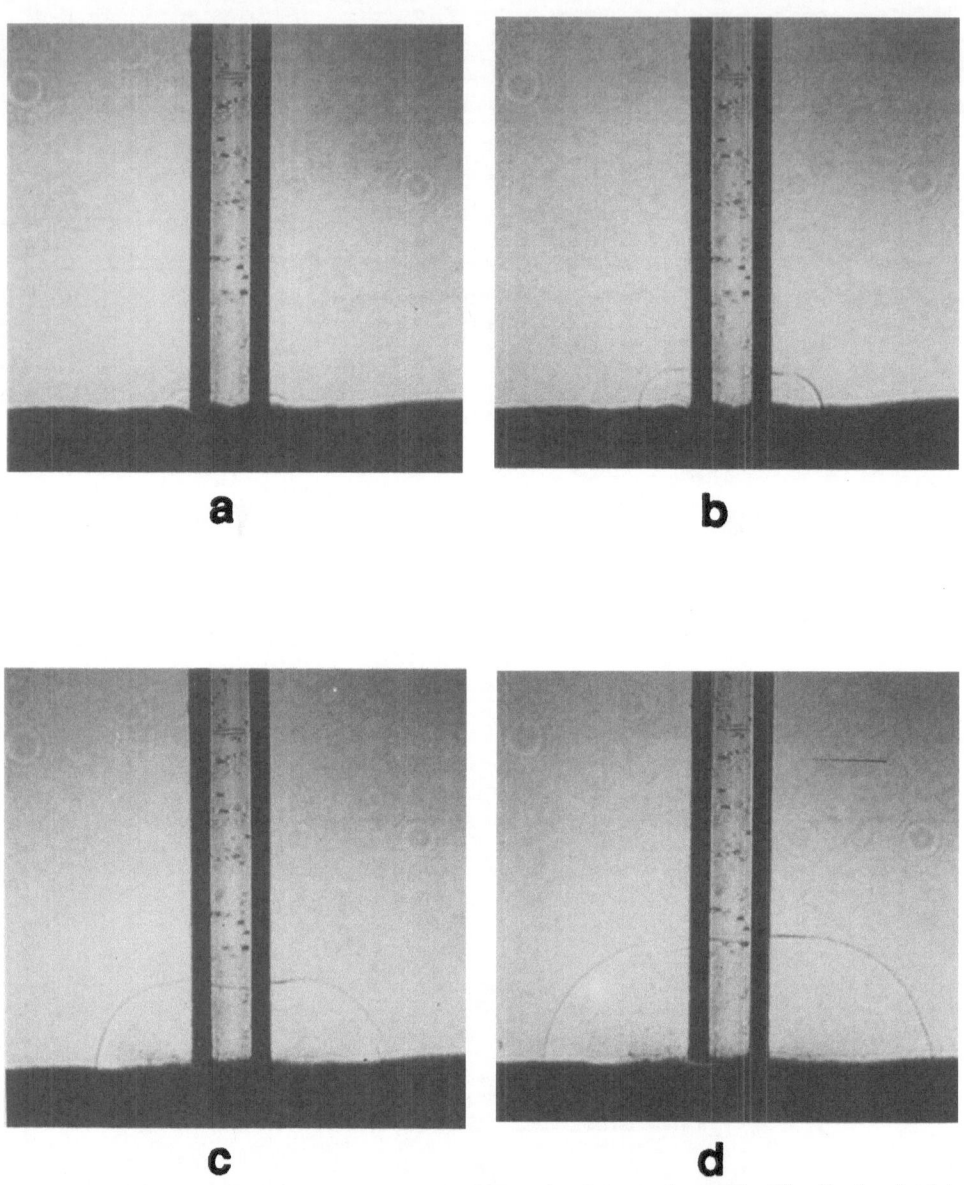

Fig. 10. Ablation of intimal wall by a single UV (308 nm) pulse seen in profile. The distal end of the fiber is just in contact with the surface of the tissue. Magnification as in Fig. 8. The delay times are: a) 250 ns, b) 500 ns, c) 1000 ns, d) 1.5 μs, e) 3 μs, f) 6 μs, g) 12 μs, and h) 18 μs.

inorganic salts appears to be the formation of pulverized particles of the salt, which are calcium phosphate (Fig. 14).

The reaction to pulverize the calcium phosphate appears to be the result of several different mechanisms which may operate in parallel. These consist of the following:
1) Although there is far less water content in the calcium phosphate than there is in the fatty part of the plaque, there is a sufficient amount for this water to be disrupted

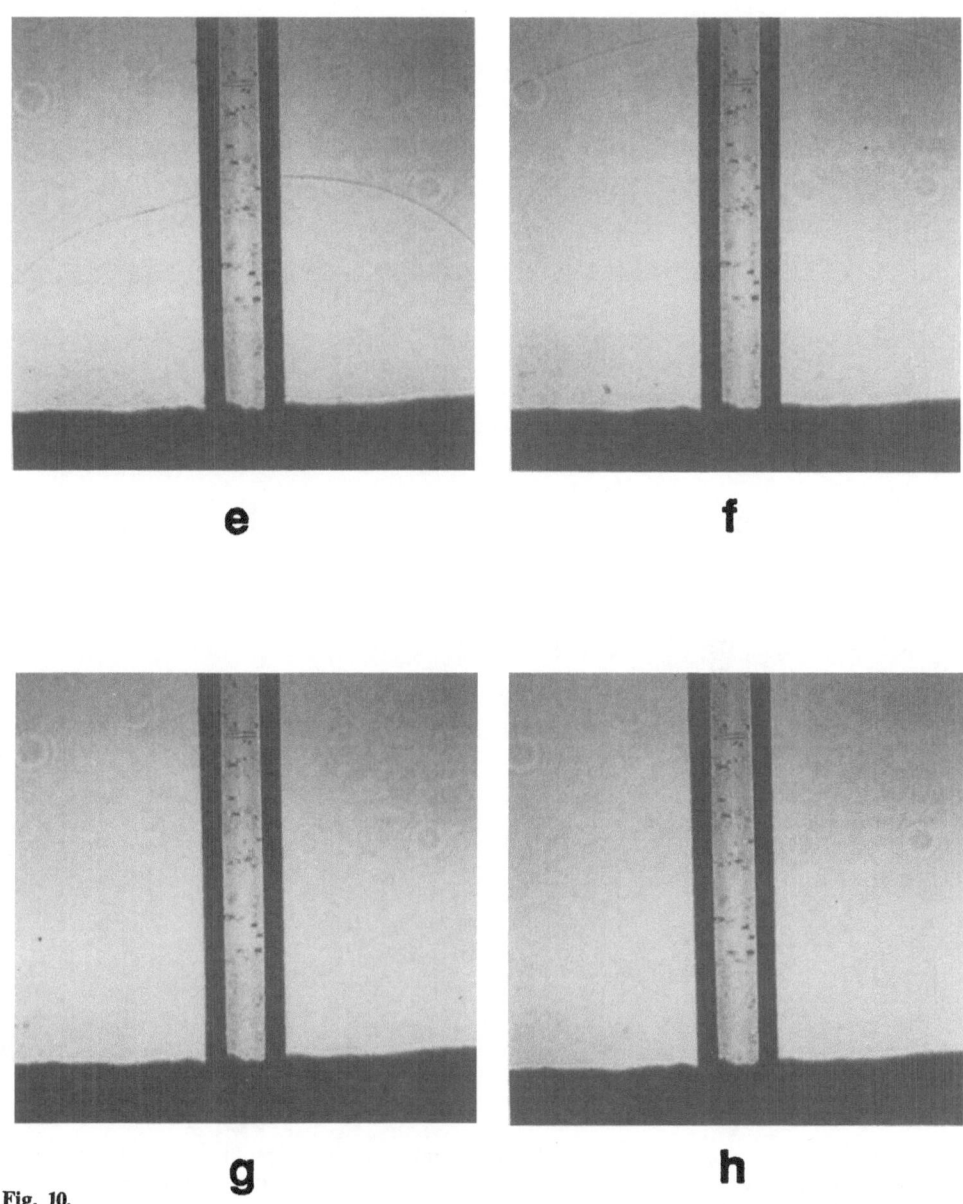

e   f

g   h

Fig. 10.

by secondary and possibly thermal means, producing steam. The steam explosion can shatter the adjacent crytalline material.

2) Absorption of the laser energy by the remaining dehydrated inorganic mineral crystals can result in differential expansion of the byproducts which, in turn, can cause shattering and disruption.

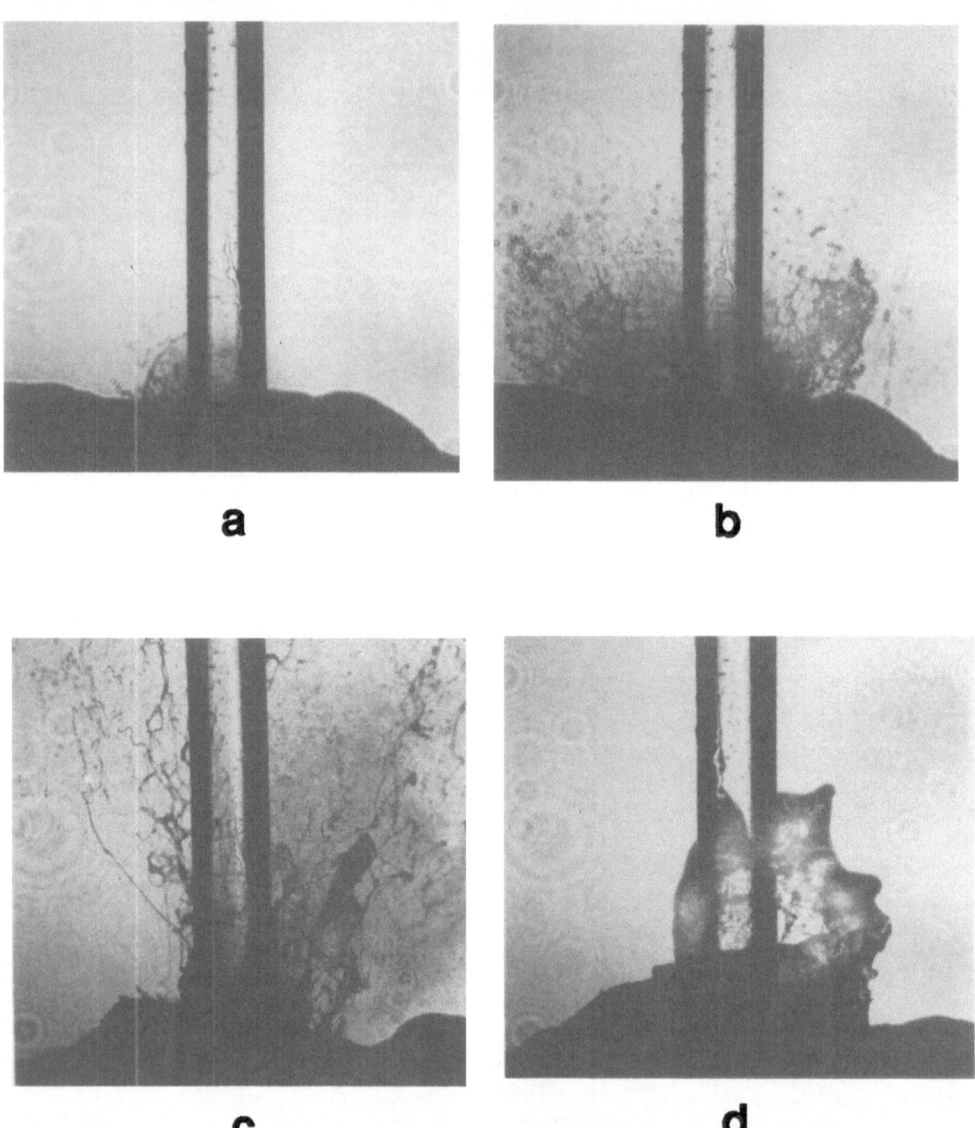

Fig. 11. Ablation of soft plaque by a single UV (308 nm) pulse seen in profile. The distal end of the fiber is just in contact with the surface of the tissue. Magnification as in Fig. 8. The delay times are: a) 6 μs, b) 15 μs, c) 30 μs, d) 60 μs, e) 100 μs, and f) ∞ time.

3) Photochemical disruption of the chemical bonds that bind the calcium phosphate molecules together is now believed to occur.
4) Mechanical vibrational disruption of the inorganic molecules has long been known in non-biologic systems. There is now both direct and indirect evidence that it occurs in the vascular system as well.
5) Release of the energy that has been stored within the inorganic plaque as it was formed. This is additional mechanical energy and possibly includes some thermal energy.

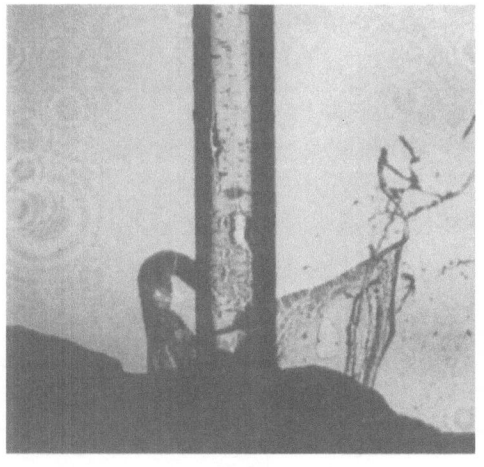
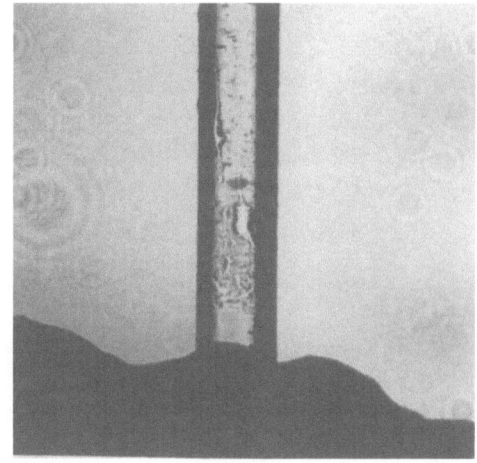

e   f

Fig. 11.

Unfortunately, laser-tissue interaction is made even more complicated by the fact that symptomatic plaque is mixed: any single spot on the target tissue may be purely inorganic or organic, but an adjacent target spot can be mixed in content. The distribution is totally random. In our own studies [18, 19], we found that virtually all human specimens of clinically significant amounts of plaque contained calcium phosphate crystals. Radiographs detected fine granules of calcium salts in most of the specimens which were thought to be free of calcium according to gross visual inspection and palpation. Energy dispersive analysis further confirmed these findings in all specimens.

Simultaneous with the efforts to develop lasers for angioplasty, efforts have continued to understand the effects of PTA/PTCA and the occurrence of restenosis. Much has been learned about the biology of this complex response to injury by the vessel wall. There are many good reviews of this important subject [20–22]. Unfortunately, there is much that is still not fully understood, and efforts to control this injury-response have not yet been successful. However, there is general agreement that myointimal hyperplasia is the final result of non-specific injury to the vessel wall, and that this biologic response results in the clinically significant restenosis of approximately 30% of successfully dilated vessels [20].

At the same time, restenosis has been noted following a variety of other mechanical debulking devices, as well as after bypass grafting with small diameter prostheses. Histopathologic studies have identified what appears to be an identical end result with intimal and smooth muscle cell hyperplasia as the cause of the obstruction [23–25].

It now appears to us that the transfer of the laser energy, which may initiate severe shock waves, may also be initiating the very same injury that has been seen with the larger, more visible tearing that results with PTA/PTCA and other mechanical devices. Evidence of deep-seated photoacoustic injury of skin from ultraviolet laser ablation

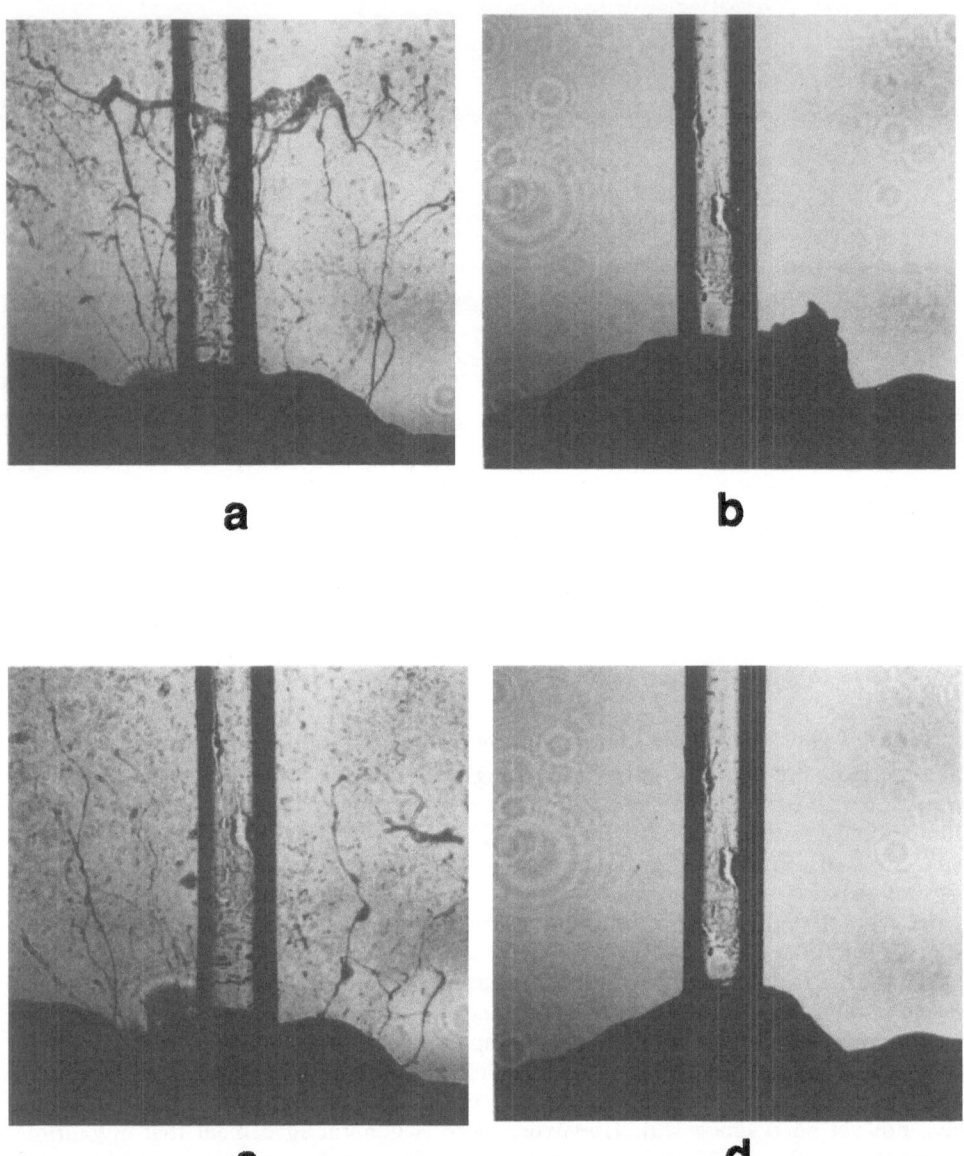

Fig. 12. Ablation of soft plaque by single UV (308 nm) pulses seen in profile. The time delay between the UV pulse and the dye laser pulse is constant at 60 µs in the four frames. a) first UV pulse on a fresh surface; b) second pulse at the same point as in a), without the fiber being advanced; c) third pulse at the same point as in a), with the fiber being advanced to make contact with the surface of the tissue; d) fourth pulse at the same point as in a) without the fiber being advanced after the third pulse.

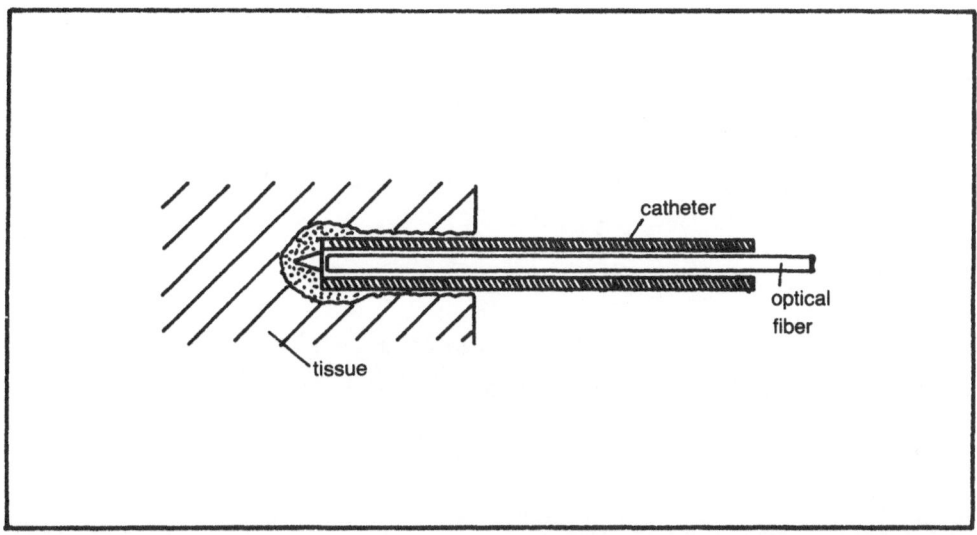

Fig. 13. Schematic diagram showing the cause of a build-up in pressure as the fiber is advanced into the tissue. As the distal end is buried into the tissue, the gases produced by the laser pulse are trapped inside the cavity that is closed off by the catheter. (Explanation based on proposal in [14].)

in experiments that were performed in vivo on an animal model has been published recently [26]. The connection, if any, between clinical results of excimer laser angioplasty in which some patients do develop restenosis, and the effect of shock waves is an extremely timely subject for investigation.

Conclusions

Pulsed, ultraviolet lasers may transfer energy at high power densities to tissue to achieve and exceed the threshold for ablation and removal of the surface layers in a controlled manner. The process is predominantly photochemical ("ablative photodecomposition") occurring at the shorter end of the ultraviolet spectrum, but introduces progressively more thermal effects as the wavelength of the laser becomes longer (but still within the UV range). Short-pulsed visible and infrared lasers produce photons of wavelengths longer than the ultraviolet. Their cutting action is entirely thermal in nature. Ablation occurs by the explosive vaporization of the water content. Pulsed infrared lasers whose wavelengths are strongly absorbed by water can be effective in tissue removal, with almost as little thermal damage as from near-ultraviolet, pulsed lasers. In all cases, pulsed lasers which operate at sufficient power densities to cause tissue ablation also cause shock waves which can injure the remaining adjacent tissue.

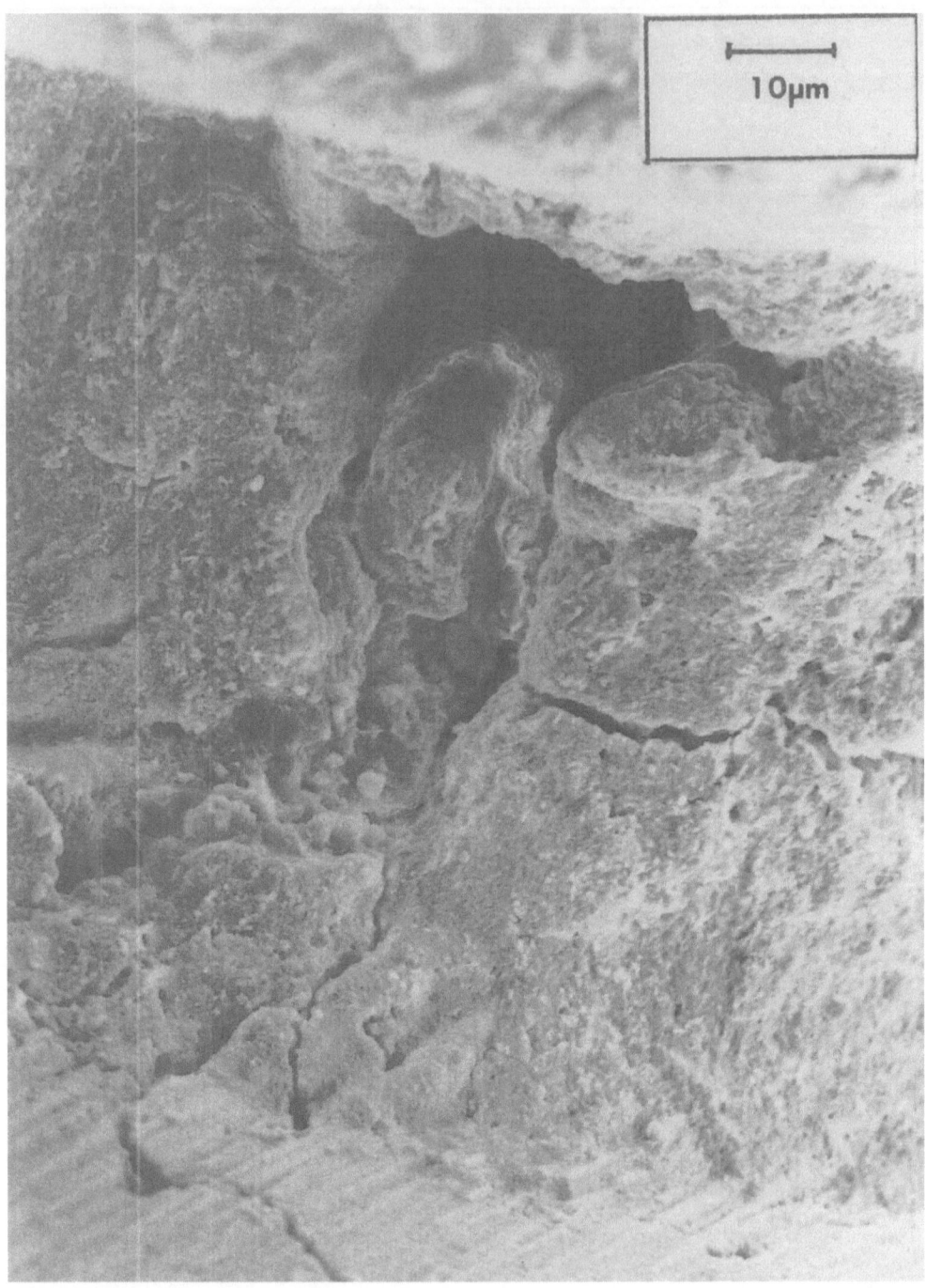

Fig. 14. Scanning electron microphotograph of hard plaque that has been shattered by exposure to UV (248 nm) laser pulses. (From [18].)

References

1. Prince MR, Deutsch TF, Mathews-Roth M, Margolis R, Parrish JA, Oseroff AR (1986) Preferential light absorption in atheromas in vitro – Implications for laser angioplasty. J Clin Invest 78: 295–302
2. Deckelbaum LI, Lam JK, Cabin HS (1987) Discrimination of normal and atherosclerotic aorta by laser-induced fluorescence. Laser Surg Med 7: 330–335
3. Prince MR, LaMuraglia GM, Teng P, Deutsch TF, Anderson RR (1987) Preferential ablation of calcified arterial plaque with laser-induced plasmas. IEEE J Quantum Elec 23: 1783–1786
4. Murphy-Chutorian D, Kosek J, Mok W, Quay S, Huestes W (1985) Selective absorption of ultraviolet laser energy by human atherosclerotic plaque treated with tetracyline. Am J Cardiol 55: 1293–1297
5. Zarins CK, Glagov S (1990) Artery wall pathology in atherosclerosis. Chap 11. Section III, in "Vascular Surgery", ed. Rutherford, RB, Saunders, Philadelphia, 3rd Ed., p. 178–193
6. Srinivasan R (1986) Ablation of polymers and biological tissue by ultraviolet lasers. Science 234: 559–565
7. Srinivasan R (1989) Laser: tissue interactions. Ber Bunsenges Phys Chem 93: 265–269
8. Srinivasan R, Wynne JJ, Blum SE (1983) Far-UV photoetching of organic material. Laser Focus 17: 62
9. Puliafito CA, Stern D, Krueger RR, Mandel ER (1987) High-speed photography of excimer laser ablation of the cornea. Arch Ophthalmology 105: 1255–1259
10. Singleton DL, Paraskevopoulos G, Jolly GS, Irwin RS, McKenney DJ (1986) Excimer lasers in cardiovascular surgery: Ablation products and photoacoustic spectrum of arterial wall. Appl Phys Lett 48: 878–880
11. Cross FW, Al-Dhahir RK, Dyer PE (1987) Ablative and acoustic response of pulsed UV laser-irradiated vascular tissue in a liquid environment. Appl Phys Lett 50: 1019
12. Bowker TJ, Cross FW, Rumsby PT, Gower MC, Rickards AF, Bown SG (1986) Excimer laser angioplasty: Quantitative comparison in vitro of three ultraviolet wavelengths on tissue ablation and haemolysis. Lasers Med Sci 1: 91–99
13. Srinivasan R, Casey KG, Haller JD (1990) Sub-nanosecond probing of the ablation of soft plaque from arterial wall by 308 nm laser pulses delivered through a fiber. IEEEJ Quantum Electronics. QE-26 Dec (in press)
14. Kar H, Biamino G (1989) Delivery systems for laser angioplasty particularly considering the safety aspects, in "Advances in Laser Medicine II". Ed.s GJ Muller and H-P Berlien, Ecomed Landsberg p.: 155–166
15. Haller JD, Krokosky EM, Srinivasan R, Wholey MH, Fisher ER (1985) Ablation of human atherosclerotic plaque by 193 and 248 nm wavelength nanosecond delivered laser energy. Proc 6th Congress, Intl Soc Laser Surg Med (Jerusalem)
16. Haller JD, Wholey MH, Fisher ER, Krokosky EM, Srinivasan R (1985) Physical and chemical effects of ultraviolet excimer laser radiation on human atherosclerotic plaque. Radiology 157: 65
17. Haller JD (1985) A sober view of laser angioplasty. Cardio 2: 31–33
18. Haller JD, Wholey MH, Fisher ER, Krokosky EM, Srinivasan R (1987) Physical and chemical effects of ultraviolet excimer laser radiation on human atherosclerotic plaque: therapeutic implications. Lasers Med Surg (Munich) 3: 98–102
19. Haller JD, Krokosky EM, Srinivasan R, Wholey MH, Fisher ER (1986) Ablation of human atherosclerotic plaque by 193 nm and 248 nm wavelength nanosecond delivered laser energy. Proc Med Biol Symp ICALEO (Toledo, OH) 49: 11
20. Liu MW, Roubin GS, King SB (1989) Restenosis after coronary angioplasty. Potential biologic determinants and role of intimal hyperplasia. Circ 79: 1374–1387
21. Painter TA (1991) Myointimal hyperplasia: Pathogenesis and implications. 1. Invitro characteristics. Artificial organs 15: 42–55
22. Macdonald RG (1990) Restenosis after PTCA. Cardio 7: 77–84
23. Garratt KN, Holmes DR Jr, Bell MR, Bresnahan JF, Kaufmann UP, Vlietstra RE, Edwards WD (1990) Restenosis after directional coronary atherectomy: Differences between primary atheromatous and restenosis lesion and influence of subintimal tissue resection. JACC 16: 1665–1671

24. Callow AD (1990) What's new in surgery: Peripheral vascular surgery. ACS bulletin 75: 49–51
25. Chervu A (1990) Myo-intimal hyperplasia. Seminars in vascular surgery 3: 21–28
26. Yashima Y, McAuliffe DJ, Jacques SL, Flotte TJ (1991) Laser-induced photoacoustic injury of skin: Effect of inertial confinement. Laser Surg Med 11: 62–68

Authors' address:
R. Srinivasan, Ph. D.
UVTech Associates
2508 Dunning Drive
Yorktown Heights
New York 10598
USA

Mid-infrared Laser Coronary Angioplasty – Experimental Study

H. J. Geschwind

Cardiac Catheterization Laboratory and Interventional Cardiology, University Hospital Henri-Mondor, INSERM U2, University Paris XII, Créteil, France

Introduction

It is well known that continuous wave lasers such as the Nd-YAG laser operating in the infrared range of wavelength allow the heat generated by the laser to diffuse away from the irradiated area, making it difficult to control ablation depth and extent of thermal necrosis. This extensive thermal injury is a significant limitation to laser application in which great precision is required, such as in the removal of atherosclerotic material from obstructed vessels [1]. Indeed, the major issue in this field is protection of the vessel wall in order to prevent perforation from occurring [2]. Over the past years there has been growing interest in using pulsed infrared lasers to ablate tissue [3, 4]. These lasers emit wavelengths that are strongly absorbed by tissue and have brief pulse durations that limit diffusion of heat from the irradiated site. Thus, they can ablate tissue while leaving only small zones of residual thermal injury. Erbium YAG and pulsed CO2 lasers are suitable for such an application, but they cannot be transmitted through currently available optical fibers, making them unsuitable for endovascular use [5].

The Holmium-YAG laser

Recently, a new laser system based on the rare earth element holmium has been developed. Its wavelenth (2.1 μm) can be transmitted through available optical fibers. It is strongly absorbed by tissue, thus producing less thermal injury than wavelengths that are poorly absorbed. The absorption coefficient of tissue at 2.1 μm is 25 cm-1, which is approximately the absorption coefficient of water. The extent of thermal injury is also determined by the thermal relaxation time of the target, which is the time required for heat to diffuse from the ablation site. Reduction of thermal damage is obtained by shortening the pulse duration of laser emission below that of relaxation time. This is the case for the Ho-YAG laser whose pulse duration is 250 μs.

Ablation mechanism

The ablation rate or the volume of tissue ablated increases linearly with delivered radiant exposure, thus allowing a precisely controlled removal of obstructing material within the arterial lumen. The irradiance capabilities are not in the range of optical breakdown and plasma formation, but are associated with a thermal mechanism causing vaporization of the target tissue. The absorption of laser irradiation and conversion into thermal

43

energy results in a local deposition of heat. As energy is added and the water in the tissue is raised to its boiling point, an explosive vaporization of the tissue will occur [6]. The dissipation of pulse energy in a thermal ablation process occurs as fire and thermal acoustic waves in a process known as spallation. Energy is dissipated in spallation through the ejection of chunks of target tissue as part of the explosive vaporization process.

Ablation characteristics

In our experimental studies, the Ho-YAG laser delivered through silica fibers was able to ablate normal, atherosclerotic and heavily calcified arterial tissue in an air or in a saline environment. However, the efficacy was higher in air (along with a deeper thermal damage) than in saline. This laser also demonstrated the ability to effectively ablate tissue in saline when the fiber tip was kept at a distance from the target tissue; this distance was shown to be below 2 mm. The energy could be transmitted through fibers as small as 100 μm, thus allowing a very flexible delivery system to be introduced into the coronary circulation.

The mechanism by which tissue is removed by this laser is explained by the two-component ablation process. In tissue such as cardiovascular obstruction the calcified deposits are not organized, but consist of salts embedded in a soft component matrix of lipids and cross-linked proteins. The soft component is vaporized readily by laser irradiation and heated fast enough to generate superheated vapor which rapidly expands, exerting force on the salt granules. The latter become dislodged and are accelerated out of the crater. Since the hot material is removed rapidly, much of the deposited heat is carried out of the crater before it can be transferred to the adjacent tissue via thermal diffusion [6].

Fiber transmission

A key factor for the effectiveness of a laser in a medical application is the laser delivery system. Because of their high transmission, light weight, small size, and flexibility, optical fibers are a very attractive delivery system for the laser. The availability of optical fibers for a particular wavelength can therefore be a critical issue in choosing the specific laser modality utilized in a medical treatment. The best optical fibers with regard to transmission, flexibility, and nontoxicity are the silica-based fibers. These fibers have excellent characteristics for wavelengths such as ruby, argon, Nd YAG, and Ho YAG. Below 400 nm, the low optical density damage threshold at these shorter wavelengths has in the past limited the use of these fibers.

Ho-YAG laser

The Ho-YAG laser is a solid-state laser whose cavity contains a Holmium-doped YAG rod optically pumped with a flashlamp [7]; it requires neither cryogenic cooling nor custom utilities. In Europe, it uses 220-volt electrical current, and has an internal water supply for cooling. It is coupled into low -OH fused silica fibers, thus differing from fibers used for Nd YAG lasers. An extremely low hydroxyl content for permits it to transmit well into the infrared.

In our laboratory, we have compared the effects on vascular tissue of various wavelengths, namely the Excimer at 308 nm, the pulsed-dye at 480 nm, and the Holmium YAG at 2.1 µm. The lasers: excimer (Spectranetics, Colorado Springs, Colorado, USA), dye (MCM, Mountain View, California) and Ho-YAG (MCM Eclipse, Mountain View, California) were coupled into single or multifiber catheters consisting of 14 to 40 fibers of 100 µm each, concentrically arranged around a central lumen for passage of a guide wire. These catheters are being currently used for clinical application in peripheral or coronary recanalization of obstructed arteries. The experimental device consisted of post mortem atherosclerotic arterial tissue which was irradiated in a saline or blood environment with the fibers maintained in a stationary position perpendicular to the target tissue. The fiber tip was either in contact with tissue or at a distance from 0.5 to 5 mm. To evaluate the true effect of laser on tissue ablation no pressure was applied at the proximal end of the catheter to be transmitted at the distal tip. Pressure waves were also measured during laser emission on tissue.

Selectivity for atheroma

The Ho-YAG laser has selectivity for atheroma ablation as compared with normal tissue. The ablation efficiency was two to three times greater for atheroma than for normal tissue. This indice of efficacy was defined as the ratio of the volume of tissue ablated by laser irradiation and the energy required. The volume of tissue ablated was measured by histologic technique and claculated from the diameter and depth of craters created into the tissue. For instance, the ablation efficiency of Ho-YAG laser irradiation was 0.05 and 0.16 mm3/Joule for normal and atherosclerotic tissue in blood medium, respectively. However, blood medium did not play a major role in the efficacy of ablation, since the figure was similar in saline. Ho-YAG was not the only one to exhibit selectivity for atheroma. This was also the case for the pulsed dye laser as opposed to the excimer laser, which did not show any preferential absorption. However, its efficiency for ablation was greater than that of the Ho-YAG even though comparison can hardly be achieved since the energy levels of the three lasers that had been evaluated were far from being similar. The only comparison that can make the study valid was due to the fact that the energies used were those routinely utilized in clinical trials and that at least for the infrared and ultraviolet laser, the study was performed with multifiber "over-the wire" catheters. It showed also that the selectivity for atheroma ablation was not decreased by saline so that no influence was exerted on the ablation characteristics of this wavelength by the commonly encountered medium circulating in vessels. The mechanism of selective ablation of atheromatous tissue could well be explained with pulsed dye laser since it is attributed to the preferential absorption of this wave length by atheroma due to the presence of carotenoid in atheromatous tissue [8]. However, such a mechanism is not likely to play a major role in the selectivity of Holmium YAG laser. It may well be due to the thermal and mechanical properties in normal and atheromatous tissue. Indeed ablation of atheroma was reported to be due, not only to vaporization, but also to liquefaction, mechanical failure, ejection of bulk material or an explosion-like process, including plasma explosion or photomechanical dissolutions. Acoustic shock or pressure waves are likely to play a role in the ablation process since they could be measured in our experimental studies. With the Holmium YAG laser the magnitude of these waves was associated with the level of ablation efficiency. They were greater for atheromatous than for normal tissue, but similar in blood and in saline. However, the ablation efficiency and the magnitude of shock waves were not related when comparing the data observed with the Ho-YAG laser with those obtained from the other sources such as excimer or pulsed dye. Indeed, the Holmium YAG laser demonstrated the greatest pressure waves and the lowest ablation efficiency. Therefore, the ablation efficiency cannot be determined only by the magnitude of shock waves, but may be due to other factors including tissue absorption coefficient.

Ablation characteristics of Ho-YAG laser

Another characteristic of the infrared laser was the ablation efficacy even when the catheter distal tip was maintained at a distance from the target. This is one of the major differences between the infrared and both the excimer and pulsed dye laser. In the latter experiments, blood attenuated the laser effects since both wavelengths are absorbed by blood. This was not the case for the Ho-YAG laser which is not absorbed to a great extent by blood medium. This finding may have major clinical implications since this is the only laser source that does not require a close contact between the site of energy delivery and the target, in other words, between the distal fiber tip and the atheromatous obstruction. This characteristic of emission may be useful in situations in which the catheter cannot be advanced against the entry of the arterial stenosis or occlusion because of narrowing of the artery.

One of the interesting observations of our studies was the diameter of craters created by the infrared laser source coupled into the multifiber catheter. The diameter of the craters was greater by 10% that of the catheter. This was not the case when pulsed dye or excimer were used. Both the Holmium YAG and the excimer laser showed a doughnut-shaped crater, as compared with the pulsed dye laser which did not exhibit any dead space or "swiss-cheese" effect in between the space not covered by the fibers. This was due to the dead space left in between the fibers. Thus, only tissue positioned in front of each distal fiber tip was ablated, whereas the running tissue located in between the fibers was not removed. A dotter effect is thought to act in dislodging this tissue during the laser procedure. The swiss-cheese effect is anticipated to be reduced once closely packed catheters are available with an increased number of fibers. Fifty fibers may be available in the near future.

Finally, all the pulsed lasers showed minimal or no thermal tissue injury as compared with continuous wave lasers. This is a major advantage for recanalization of obstructed coronary or peripheral arteries.

Clinical implications

In summary, the experimental studies on laser angioplasty using a mid-infrared source such as the Holmium YAG suggest some advantages over other wavelengths that are currently being used in clinical trials. These include the ability to act at a distance from the target, which implies an adequate transmission through blood. The clinical implication is the possibility for the distal laser catheter tip not to be positioned in close contact with the arterial obstruction. We could anticipate that an irradiating laser at a distance from the target could allow the diverging light to create larger crater diameters than those obtained with the fibers in contact with tissue. In such a position, even a divergent beam would hardly allow the light to diverge through the tissue. The preferential absorption by atheromatous tissue, as demonstrated by a lower energy threshold and a greater ablation efficiency, is likely to increase both the efficacy and the safety of the procedure. The procedure is anticipated to be more effective because the ablation efficiency demonstrated by in vitro studies is greater in atheroma than in healthy tissue. The safety is likely to be increased since the ablation energy threshold can be decreased, allowing atheromatous but not healthy tissue to be ablated.

In contrast, two effects could be deleterious. Thermal damage to the surrounding tissue was shown in our studies to expand slightly beyond that observed with the excimer laser. Furthermore, the high energy level required for ablation may induce pressure or acoustic shock waves, which were shown in our studies to be 10 to 20 times greater than those measured with excimer lasers. The clinical consequences of this mechanical effect have not been precisely evaluated and deserve further study.

References

1. Isner JM, Donaldson RF, Deckelbaum LI, Clarke RH, Laliberte SM, Ucci AA, Salem DN, Kostam MA (1985) The excimer laser: gross, light microscopic and ultrastructural analysis of potential advantages for use in laser therapy of cardiovascular disease. J Am Coll Cardiol 6: 1102–1109
2. Grundfest WS, Litvack F, Forrester JS, Goldenberg T, Swan HJC, Morgenstern L, Fishbein M, Mc Dermid IS, Rider DM, Pascala TJ, Laudenslader JB (1985) Laser ablation of human atherosclerotic plaque without adjacent tissue injury. J Am Coll Cardiol 5: 929–933
3. Treat MR, Trokel SL, Reynolds D, DeFilippi VJ, Andrew J, Ying Liu J, Cohen MG (1988) Preliminary evelution of a pulsed 2.15-μm laser system for fiberoptic endoscopic surgery. Lasers Surg Med 8: 322–326
4. Aretz HT, Butterly JR, Jewell ER, Setzer SE, Shapsey SM (1989) Effects of holmium-YSGG laser irradiation on arterial tissue: preliminary results. SPIE 1067: 127–132
5. Charlton A, Dickinson MR, King TA, Freemont AJ (1990) Erbium YAG and Holmium YAG laser ablation of bone. Lasers Med Science 5: 365–373
6. Izatt JA, Albagli D, Itzkan I, Feld MS (1990) Pulsed laser ablation of clacified tissue: physical mechanism and fundamental parameters. SPIE 1202: 133–140
7. Nuss RC, Fabian RL, Sarkar R, Puliafito CA (1988) Infrared laser bone ablation. Lasers Surg Med 8: 381–391
8. Prince MR, Deutsch TF, Mathews-Roth MM, Margolis R, Parrish JA, Oseroff AR (1986) Preferential light absorption in atheromas in vitro. Implication for laser angioplasty. J Clin Invest 78: 295–302

Authors address:
Herbert J. Geschwind, M. D., FACC
Chu Henri Mondor
51, av. du Marechal de Lattre de Tassigny
F-94010 Créteil
France

Time-Course of Smooth Muscle Cell Proliferation following Balloon Angioplasty and Excimer Laser Treatment in an Experimental Animal Model

H. Hanke, K. K. Haase, M. Oberhoff, and K. R. Karsch

Division of Cardiology, Department of Medicine, University of Tübingen, FRG

Introduction

Since Grüntzig et al. [2] introduced Percutaneous Transluminal Coronary Angioplasty (PTCA) in 1977, this technique has become a successful method in the treatment of patients with coronary artery disease [3]. The clinical application of PTCA, however, is limited by the occurrence of restenosis in 30–40% of primary successful treated patients [4, 5, 6]. Transluminal angioplasty, performed with an inflatable balloon, is associated with endothelial denudation and early accumulation of platelets and fibrin [7, 8], splitting of the intima and media [9–11], stretching of the medial layer, and overdistention of the adventitia [12, 13]. Platelet adhesion and aggregation induced by endothelial injury following balloon angioplasty has been shown to result in the release of several mitogens [14], including epidermal growth factor (EGF) and platelet-derived growth factor (PDGF). These components, as well as expression of fibroblast growth factor (FGF) and activation of macrophages, are thought to stimulate migration and proliferation of smooth muscle cells (SMC) in the dilated artery [15–18]. In addition, stimulated smooth muscle cells are also capable of producing intrinsic growth factors [19]. Smooth muscle cell proliferation following PTCA was found to be important for the development of restenosis in several experimental and human postmortem studies [20–22].

To improve the long-term efficacy for treatment of coronary artery disease, the application of laser systems for the removal of atherosclerotic artery obstructions has been suggested as an alternative method [23–25].

However, application of thermal lasers (i. e., argon, carbon dioxide, or Nd:YAG) is limited, due to coagulation, necrosis of vascular tissue, perforation, and thrombosis [26–28]. In contrast, experimental in vitro and in vivo studies have demonstrated that XeCl excimer lasers can perform efficient tissue microablation with only minimal thermal injury of adjacent tissue [11, 29, 30]. The ablative mechanism of excimer lasers is supposed to be based on "ablative photodecomposition" and a generation of pressure waves resulting in fragmentation of tissue structures [31].

The current clinical results suggest that excimer laser angioplasty may become an alternative or adjunctive treatment for patients with coronary artery disease [32–35].

Thus, the rationale of this experimental study was to determine the temporal sequence of morphological changes after conventional balloon dilatation and after excimer laser ablation in the identical model of atherosclerotic rabbit carotid arteries. In addition, the extent of mitosis of vascular smooth muscle cells was determined at different time intervals following balloon and laser treatment by bromodeoxyuridine-labeling.

49

Methods

Animal model

Fibromuscular plaques were produced before balloon and laser treatment using the electrostimulation method as described by Betz and Schlote [36].

For implantation of two graphite-coated gold electrodes at the carotid artery, 84 male New Zealand rabbits were anesthetized with intramuscular injections of 8 mg metomidate-HCl and 0.1 mg fentanyl-base/kg b. wt. After preparation of the right carotid artery the electrodes were diametrically attached to the adventitia and held in position by an 8-mm-long teflon-cuff. Thin subcutaneously placed leads were connected to a small plastic socket fixed at the skull. Connecting an external stimulation unit to the socket, constant-current DC impulses (15 ms/imp., 0.1 mA, Hz) were transmurally applied twice daily in the carotid artery of each animal for 30 min in the morning and 15 min in the afternoon with a time interval of 8–10 h between the stimulation cycles. This protocol was carried out for 28 days. In order to produce atheromatous plaques by electrical stimulation the animals were additionally fed with a commercially avaiable 0.5% cholesterol diet (Altromin, Lage, FRG) during the stimulation period [37, 38].

Study protocol

Balloon angioplasty

After 28 days of electrical stimulation the animals were separated into two groups.

Balloon dilatation was performed in 35 rabbits under general anesthesia. After preparation of the carotid artery, the exposed vessel was ligated at least 3-cm distal from the implanted electrodes. Angioplasty was performed with a 2.0-mm balloon-catheter (Micro-Hartzler, ACS, California, USA) which was introduced by direct arteriotomy, then advanced into the region of the plaque under microscopic control. The angioplasty catheter was inflated two times with 5 atm for 30 s. Between the two dilatations the balloon was deflated for 30 s. After removal of the deflated catheter, the small incision of the arteriotomy was closed and arterial blood flow restored. To avoid bacterial infections, all animals were on antibiotic therapy for 3 days following the procedure. Standard heparin was not administered during or after intervention. After balloon angioplasty a commercially available standard diet without cholesterol (Fa. Altromin) was fed.

To study the time-course of SMC proliferation and the chronological sequence of morphological changes, the animals were sacrificed 3, 7, 14, 21, 28 days, and 6 weeks after transluminal balloon angioplasty. A minimum of five animals was used in each group. Ten control animals were separated into two groups of five rabbits each. One group of rabbits was electrically stimulated for 28 days and served as a control group without angioplasty. Five other rabbits were used as sham controls to exclude an additional effect on SMC proliferation during the mechanical placement of the catheter. The animals in the sham-operated group underwent a stimulation period of 28 days; arteriotomy without inserting the catheter was performed. These animals were sacrificed 7 days after intervention.

50

Excimer laser angioplasty

Laser system and catheter device: A commercial xenon chloride excimer laser (MAX-10, Technolas Inc., Munich) emitting light at a wavelength of 308 nm with a pulse duration of 60 ns was used. The laser was operated at a repetition rate of 20 Hz. The laser beam was focused into a cathether device consisting of 20 quartz fibers of 100 μm core diameter each. The transmitted energy densities were measured before and after treatment with a conventional power meter and were, with 40 mJ/mm², above the ablation threshold.

The fiberoptic quartz fibers were arranged concentrically around a central lumen suitable for a 0.014 inch guide wire and fixed only at the proximal and distal ends, to ensure maximal catheter shaft flexibility. The cross-sectional diameter of the catheter device was 1.3 mm.

Experimental laser ablation: After 28 days of electrical stimulation, 39 rabbits were anesthetized, and after preparation of the right carotid artery the exposed vessel was ligated by two clamps. Transversal arteriotomy was subsequently performed between the two clamps. The carotid artery and the exposed lumen surface was kept moist with 0.9% NaCl solution during the whole procedure.

The laser catheter was inserted into the lumen of the artery under microscopic control. After removal of the cranial clamp the catheter was manually advanced to the region of plaque. Excimer laser energy was applied while the catheter tip was slowly (4 mm in 15 s) advanced into the region of plaque, beginning 4 mm caudal, and terminated 4 mm cranial of the implanted electrodes. Additional ablation was performed during withdrawal (16 mm in 20 s) of the catheter. After a second advance and withdrawal (each performed with a speed of 16 mm in 20 s) by continuous energy delivery the laser catheter was removed. The cranial artery clamp was subsequently replaced. In order to reestablish arterial blood flow the arteriotomy was closed with a 7-0 polypropylene suture. To avoid bacterial infections, all animals were on antibiotic therapy during the following 3 days. To reduce acute mural thrombus formation, a bolus of 700 I. E./kg b. wt. standard heparin was given subcutaneously at 2 h before laser treatment. In addition, all animals received 900 I. E./kg b. wt. s. c. twice daily for 72 h after laser ablation. The cholesterol-containing diet was not continued and all animals received a standard diet (Altromin, Lage, FRG).

To compare the temporal sequence of morphological changes and SMC proliferation in the balloon-dilated animals, the laser-treated vessels were also excised after 3, 7, 14, 21, 28, and 42 days following intervention.

Five other animals were used as sham controls in order to assess a possible mechanical injury derived from the catheter during the laser treatment procedure. The animals in the sham-operated group, which had also received electrostimulation for 28 days, underwent arteriotomy and insertion of the catheter without application of laser energy. All these animals were sacrificed 7 days after the procedure.

Tissue analysis

Application of bromodeoxyuridine

Bromodeoxyuridine-labeling was performed in all animals to determine the number of smooth muscle cells undergoing DNA synthesis at different time intervals after balloon and laser treatment.

As described previously [38, 39], 100 mg bromodeoxyuridine (BrdU)/kg b. wt. and 75 mg deoxycytidine (d-cyt)/kg b. wt. were given as a subcutaneous neck, depot 18 h before the animals were sacrificed. In addition, intramuscular injections (30 mg BrdU/kg b. wt. and 25 mg d.cyt/kg b. wt.) 18 h and 12 h before perfusion fixation were given.

Perfusion fixation

After application of an overdose of metomidate-HCl and fentanyl-base, thoracotomy was performed. The carotid arteries were fixed in situ with perfusion of 500 ml 0.1 M cacodylate-buffered 2% paraformaldehyde solution at a pressure of 60–80 mmHg via a catheter inserted into the left ventricle.

The excised vessels were immersion-fixed in 2% cacodylate-buffered paraformaldehyde for at least 6 h.

Histological examination

The arterial segments below the teflon-cuff were used for histological analysis. The excised samples were embedded in paraffin and prepared for histological and immunohistological examination.

The embedded arterial segments were cut into a series beginning at the caudal end of the balloon/laser-treated region to the maximal extent of plaque. The 4-μm-thin cross-sections were then used for histological and immunohistological analysis. Standard hemalaune, hematoxylin, and eosin strains were prepared; stained sections were evaluated with respect to the extent of intimal hyperplasia, intimal dissection, and laser-specific alterations such as vacuolization, carbonization, and intimal fissuring. Local reduction of SMC nuclei as observed after excimer laser ablation in the media was qualitatively determined.

The extent of intimal cell layers was determined by counting the number of cell nuclei on the perpendicular line between endothelium and internal elastic membrane at the area of maximal plaque size. Animals with evidence of thrombus formation were excluded from this analysis.

The immunohistological quantification of cells undergoing DNA synthesis was previously described [38] and is based on staining (biotin-avidin method [40, 41]) with a monoclonal antibody against bromodeoxyuridine (Bio Cell Consulting, Grellingen, Switzerland). This technique allows identification of all proliferated cells, which entered s-phase during the 18 h of the labeling period. In addition, immunohistochemical detection (FITC-labeled immunofluorescence (Sigma GmbH, Deisenhofen, FRG) and avidin biotin method) of the alpha-SM isoform of actin (monoclonal antibody from Renner, Dannstadt, FRG) was performed to identify the neointimal proliferated cells as SMCs.

All BrdU-positive cells and the total number of cells were separately counted in the intimal and medial cross-sectional area as previously described [38, 42]. The proliferative response of SMC following balloon and laser treatment was calculated as the relation of BrdU-positive cells to the total cell number expressed in percent for both layers separately.

Statistical evaluation

All values are expressed as mean ± standard deviation (SD). The statistical significance of differences between control and balloon – or laser-treated arteries were determined using twotailed Student's t-test. Differences were considered significant if $p < 0.05$ (43).

Results

Morphological results following balloon angioplasty

After 28 days of electrical stimulation, microscopic examination showed a plaque located beneath the anode of the electrode in control animals (Fig. 1). The endothelial lining was intact and quantification of intimal SMC layers in the region of maximal plaque size displayed a mean of 13 ± 5 cell layers in the control vessels. Figure 2 shows a progressive and continuous increase of intimal thickening in all dilated arteries from 13 ± 5 cell layers of the electrically stimulated control group, to 33 ± 14 cell layers after 4 weeks following angioplasty ($p < 0.05$, t-test). However, later than 4 weeks after angioplasty no additional increase of the number of intimal SMC layers occurred. Histological examination revealed a stenosis of more than 50% of lumen diameter due to an intimal hyperplasia in three of 35 animals (Table 1). In these cases an excessive proliferation of SMC was observed (Fig. 3). Focal intimal dissection or medial disrupture was not found in these segments. In five other animals a complete thrombotic occlusion was found. The mural thrombi observed after angioplasty showed evidence of fibromuscular organization and all of these thrombi were partially recanalized. Medial disrupture was seen in two other animals and both were associated with mural thrombi reducing the luminal diameter by less than 50%. In four dilated arteries a focal splitting of the intima with shearing off of the endothelial layer was observed.

Quantification of SMC proliferation following balloon angioplasty after labeling with BrdU.

In control animals without angioplasty, quantification of intimal and medial SMC proliferation showed no statistical differences between the normal (intima: $0.9 \pm 0.5\%$, media: $0.4 \pm 0.3\%$) and the sham-operated group (intima: $0.7 \pm 0.6\%$, media: $0.3 \pm 0.2\%$).

A total of 30 dilated arteries was used for determination of SMC proliferation. Animals with evidence of mural thrombi were excluded from SMC analysis. Quantification of intimal SMC proliferation revealed a significant increased number of cells undergoing DNA synthesis at 3 ($9.6 \pm 4.6\%$) and 7 days ($8.4 \pm 4.4\%$) after angioplasty

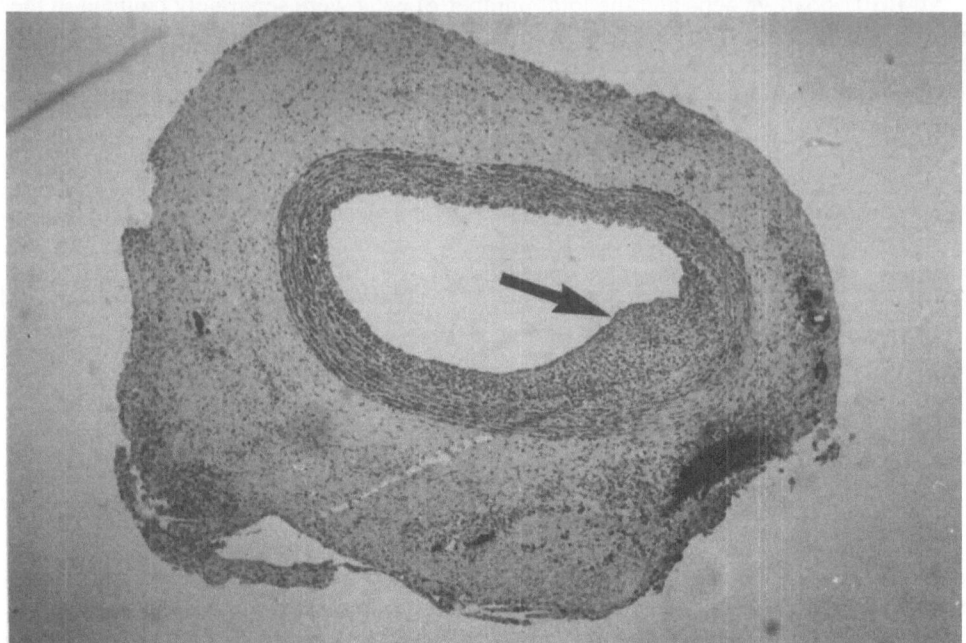

Fig. 1. Light micrograph of a rabbit carotid artery after 28 days of electrical stimulation (paraffin-embedding). Concentric fibromuscular proliferation in the intima with a maximum of plaque size (arrow) below the graphite-coated electrode (anode). Magnification × 12.5; Hemalaune combined with immunohistological staining of alpha-actin (avidin biotin).

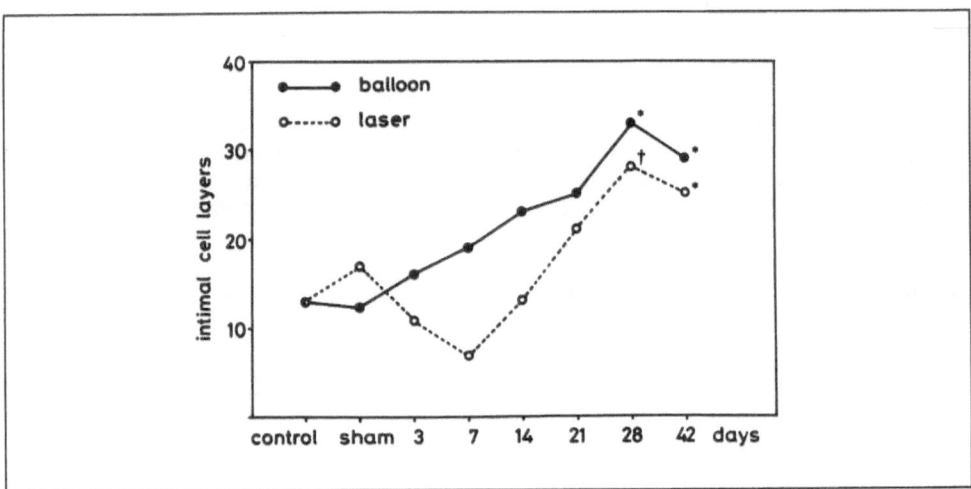

Fig. 2. Quantification of intimal cell layers (SMC) following transluminal balloon angioplasty and excimer laser ablation in 68 treated carotid arteries after immunohistological staining of alpha-actin. Note standard deviation of each in Tables 1 Table 2. (*$p < 0.05$, †$p < 0.01$ compared to control animals).

Table 1. Histomorphological and immunohistological findings following transluminal balloon angioplasty. All values are expressed in mean ±SD.

Study group	Animals (No. 1)	Stenosis >50% by SMCs	Stenosis >50% by thrombus	Intimal SMC-layers [× + SD]	Intimal BrdU-labeled cells [%, × + SD]	Medial BrdU-labeled cells [%, × + SD]
Control	5	0/5	0/5	13± 5	0.9±0.5	0.4±0.3
Sham-operated	5	0/5	0/5	12± 4	0.7±0.6	0.3±0.2
3 days	5	0/5	0/5	16± 9	9.6±4.6†	1.3±1.8
7 days	6	0/6	1/6	19± 9	8.4±4.4†	2.1±2.1
14 days	6	0/6	1/6	23± 9	1.2±0.5	1.1±1.0
21 days	7	1/7	2/7	25±18	1.2±0.5	2.1±1.6*
28 days	6	1/6	1/6	33±14*	0.3±0.2	0.5±0.4
42 days	5	1/5	0/5	29+14*	0.2+0.1	0.3+0.2

* statistically significant compared to control group ($p < 0.05$, t-test)
† statistically significant compared to control group ($p < 0.01$, t-test)

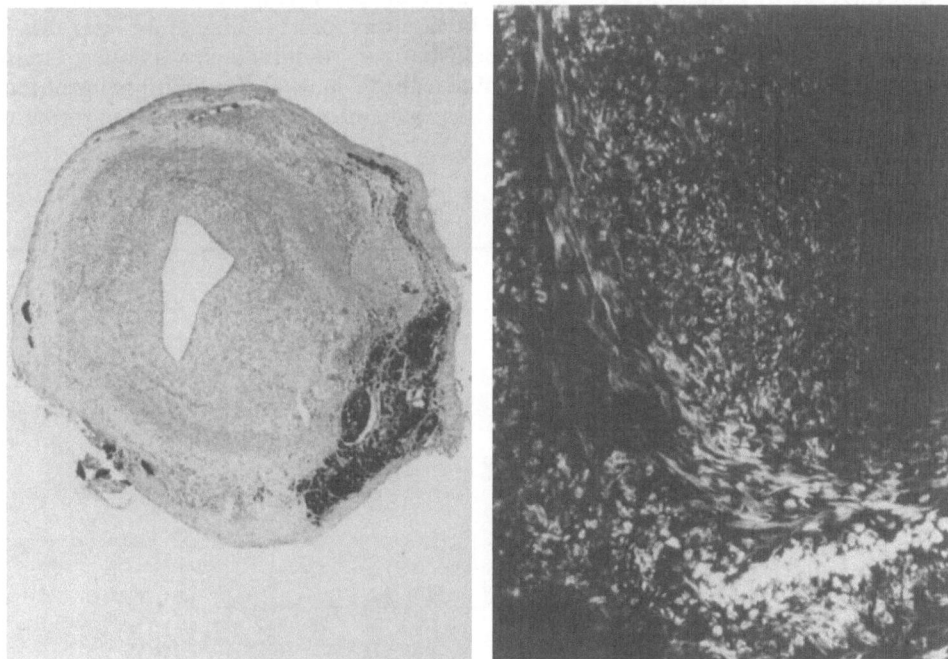

Fig. 3. Cross-section of a dilated artery 21 days after balloon treatment.
Panel A: Significant stenosis at the site of dilatation (magnification × 12.5, hematoxylin and eosin staining)
Panel B: Histological section of the same lesion (magnification × 78) showing that stenosis is mainly due to intimal proliferation of SMC (FITC—labeled immunofluorescence of alpha-actin, as a smooth muscle specific marker).

55

(p < 0.01) and a decrease of proliferation between days 7 and 14 following intervention (Figs. 4 and 5).

In contrast to the intimal SMC proliferation, medial SMC proliferation was moderate and had a small but significant increase of cells undergoing DNA synthesis at 21 days (p < 0.05) after angioplasty (Fig. 4). Twenty-eight days after dilatation the extent of SMC undergoing DNA synthesis in the media and intima was normalized and reached the values of pre-intervention measurement.

Morphological results following excimer laser angioplasty

In the sham-operated control group intimal proliferation of SMC resulted in a fibromuscular plaque consisting of 17 ± 7 cell layers at 7 days after intervention. The difference compared to the control group (see above) was not statistically significant.

Determination of the maximum number of intimal SMC layers showed an intimal wall thickness of 11 ± 7 cell layers after 3 days, and of 7 ± 6 cell layers after 7 days following laser treatment. After 7 days, a continuous increase of intimal SMC layers was found during the following 3 weeks. After 28 days mean intimal wall thickness was 28 ± 5 cell layers and was statistically significantly different from the control group without laser ablation (p < 0.01). Forty-two days after treatment, however, no additional increase of intimal plaque size could be observed (Fig. 2).

A stenosis of more than 50% luminal reduction was found in nine of 34 laser-treated arteries (26%). In four rabbits a total occlusion was found which was due to mural thrombus formation. In four of the nine animals the lesion was due to intimal proliferation of SMCs (Fig. 6), and in one artery a partial fibromuscular organized thrombus

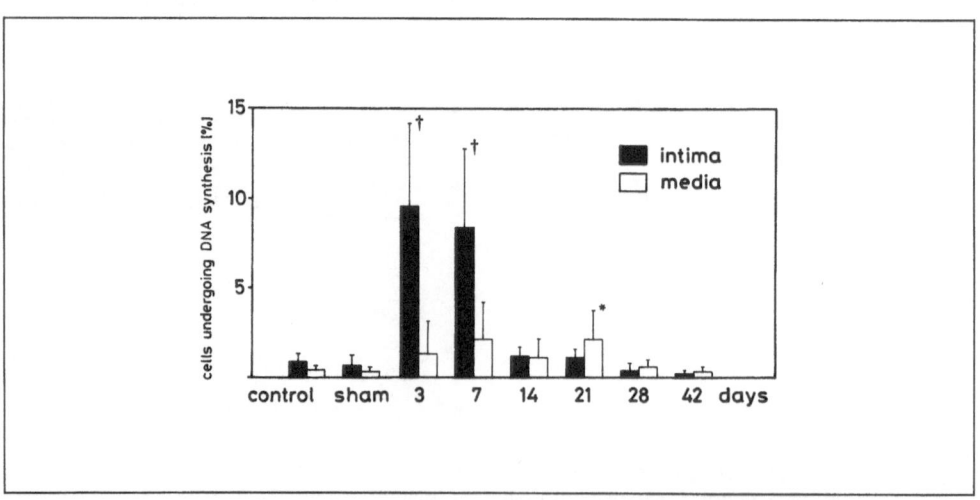

Fig. 4. Time-course of intimal and medial SMC undergoing DNA synthesis following angioplasty. Shown are the results of 30 dilated arteries after labeling with bromodeoxyuridine. Values are expressed as mean ± SD from five animals in each dilated group (*p < 0.05, †p < 0.01 compared to control group).

56

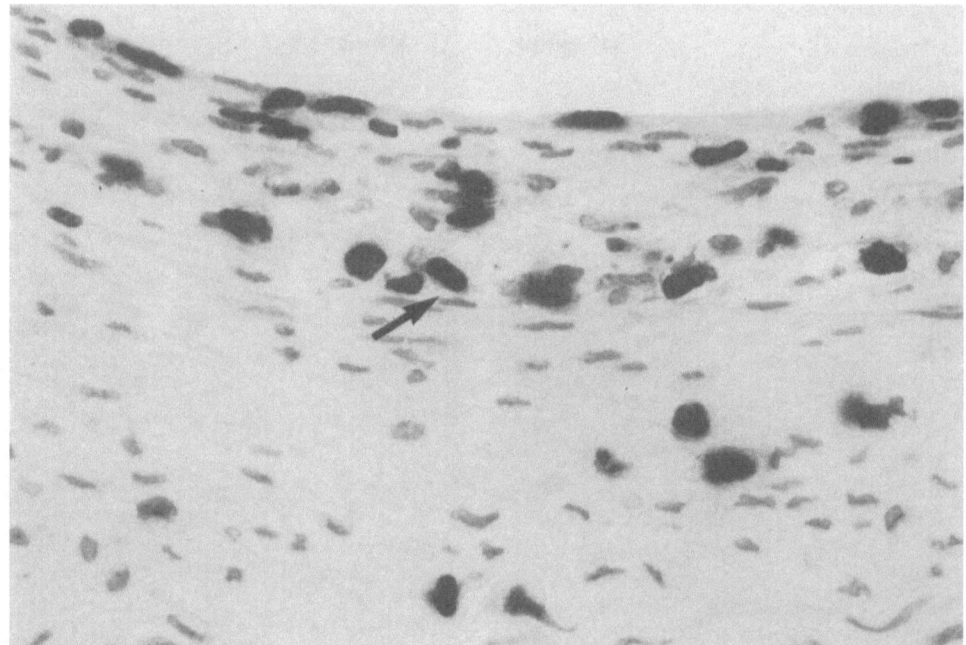

Fig. 5. Histological section of carotid artery at 7 days after transluminal angioplasty. Avidin biotin staining of BrdU shows a large number of labeled cells (arrow) in the intimal proliferate (magnification × 188).

and additional considerable intimal SMC proliferation was found. In addition, mural thrombus formation resulting in a stenosis <50% was found in two arteries.

Evidence of vacuoules in the intimal layer was observed in 10 vessels. No vessel perforation occurred, but tissue ablation into the medial layer was found in 12 arteries. In 10 of these arteries, ablation was associated with a local reduction of SMCs in the media (Fig. 7). In the residual two animals with ablation of the medial tissue this phenomenon was not observed (Table 2). However, evidence for carbonization and intimal fissuring was not found in any artery.

Quantification of SMC proliferation following excimer laser angioplasty after labeling with BrdU

Calculation of cells undergoing DNA synthesis in the sham-operated animals showed no statistically significant differences in regard to SMC proliferation in the intimal and medial layers compared to the electrically stimulated control group.

As shown in Fig. 8, quantification of intimal SMC proliferation revealed a significant increase of cells entering s-phase of mitosis during the first 14 days after excimer laser ablation (3 days: $2.9 \pm 1.7\%$, $p < 0.05$, 7 days: $5.9 \pm 6.1\%$, $p < 0.25$ (n. s.), 14 days: $5.6 \pm 2.3\%$, $p < 0.01$). Twenty-one days after laser treatment the extent of cells undergoing DNA synthesis was decreased and comparable to the control and sham-operated group. In contrast to the intimal proliferation, the mean percentage of cells

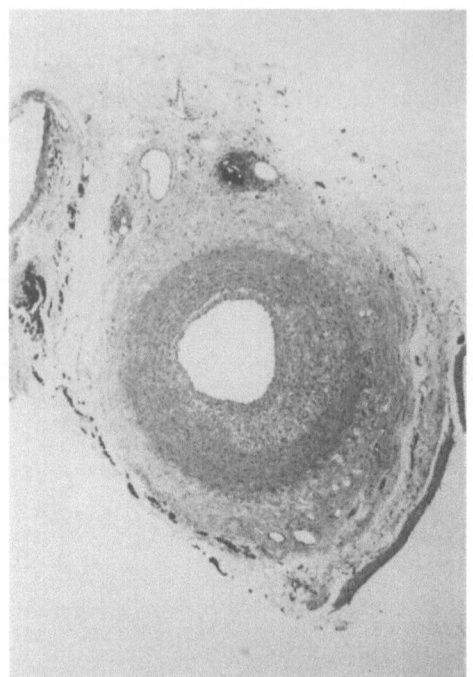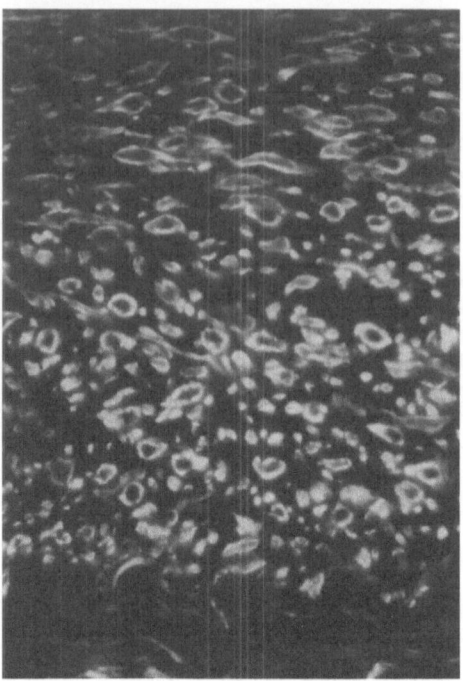

Fig. 6. Cross-section of a laser-treated artery 28 days after excimer laser ablation
Panel A: Intimal thickening with significant reduction of the cross-sectional lumen area (magnification × 12.5, hematoxylin and eosin staining).
Panel B: Histological section of the same vessel with a higher magnification (× 125), demonstrating that the stenosis is predominately due to intimal proliferation of SMCs (fluorescein isothiocyanate-labeled immunofluorescence of alpha actin).

entering s-phase of mitosis in the media was only moderately increased, and had a small but significant increase of mitosis at 7 days ($p < 0.05$) after intervention. Twenty-eight days after laser treatment the extent of cells which had synthesized DNA in both layers was normalized.

Discussion

The early and late morphological changes after transluminal angioplasty have been reported in several experimental and postmortem studies, but little is known about the dynamic process of cellular proliferation and its implication for the development of restenosis following PTCA or excimer laser treatment [20–22, 44, 45].

Animal model

It is extremly difficult to find an appropriate animal model of advanced atherosclerosis and, therefore, all experimental studies are limited and cannot be transferred to the situation in humans.

58

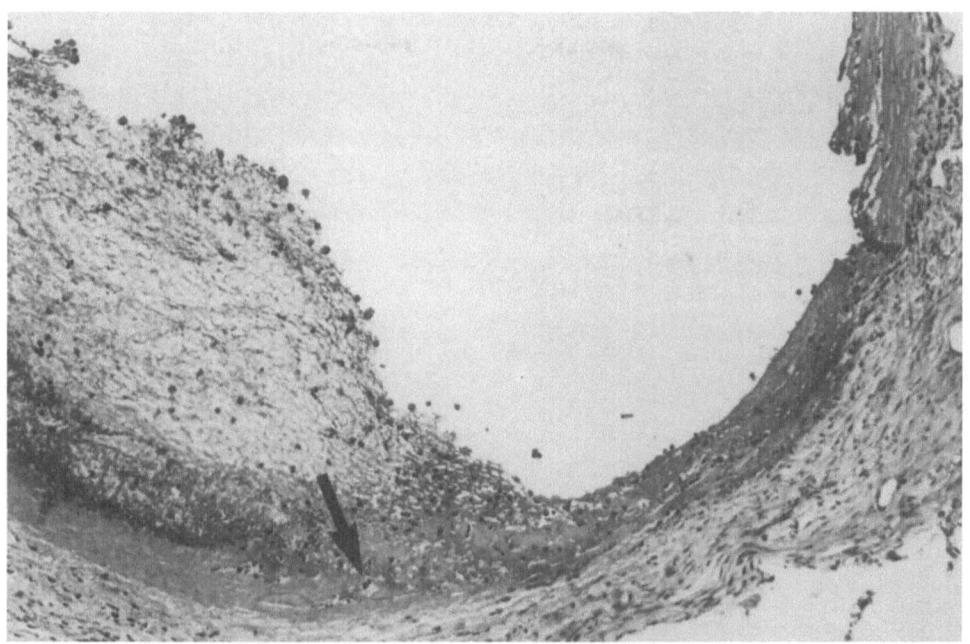

Fig. 7. Histological cross-section 3 days after excimer laser treatment (magnification × 40, hematoxylin and eosin staining). Tissue ablation in the media (arrow) resulted in local thrombus formation and reduction of SMC nuclei in the media.

A high-cholesterol diet, which is important for the production of an atheroma after local endothelial denudation with a balloon, induces very high serum levels of cholesterol and is associated with a larger number of foam cells in the neo-intima [46]. Endothelial denudation by balloon injury leads, however, to damage of the natural endothelial layer [47, 48]. Especially in this model it might be difficult to differentiate the effects of angioplasty from the effect of primary injury.

The advantage of the model of electrical stimulation in producing atherosclerotic lesions is the induction of fibromuscular plaques of comparable size under standardized conditions while maintaining the integrity of the endothelial layer [49, 50]. This fibromuscular plaque might be comparable to the early stage of atherosclerotic lesions in humans [51, 52].

This model, however, is limited since it is impossible to induce a high-degree stenosis or even subtotal lesion in rabbit carotid arteries.

Experimental balloon angioplasty

Quantification of SMC proliferation in the sham-operated and control animals without balloon angioplasty showed no statistical difference, demonstrating that the increase in DNA synthesis of SMC following angioplasty was due to the effect of balloon treatment only. Furthermore, our results demonstrate that intimal SMC proliferation is a

Table 2. Histomorphological and immunohistological findings following excimer laser treatment. All values are expressed in mean ±SD.

Study group	Animals (No.)	Stenosis >50% by SMCs	Stenosis >50% by thrombus	Intimal SMC-layers [$\times + SD$]	Ablation into the media	Medial SMC reduction	Intimal BrdU-labeled cells [%, $\times + SD$]	Medial BrdU-labeled cells [%, $\times + SD$]
Sham-operated	5	1/5	0/5	17±7	0/5	0/5	1.0±0.5	0.7±0.5
3 days	7	1/7	2/7	11±7	4/7	4/7	2.9±1.7*	2.2±2.1
7 days	7	0/7	0/7	7±6	1/7	3/7	5.9±6.1	3.9±3.3*
14 days	5	0/5	1/5	13±7	1/5	3/5	5.3±2.3†	1.3±0.7
21 days	5	2/5	0/5	21±8	2/5	1/5	1.6±1.4	0.9±0.5
28 days	5	1/5	0/5	28±5†	2/5	2/5	0.6±0.5	0.7±0.8
42 days	5	1/5	1/5	23±5*	2/5	2/5	0.5±0.4	0.5±0.2

* statistically significant compared to control group ($p < 0.05$, t-test)
† statistically significant compared to control group ($p < 0.01$, t-test)

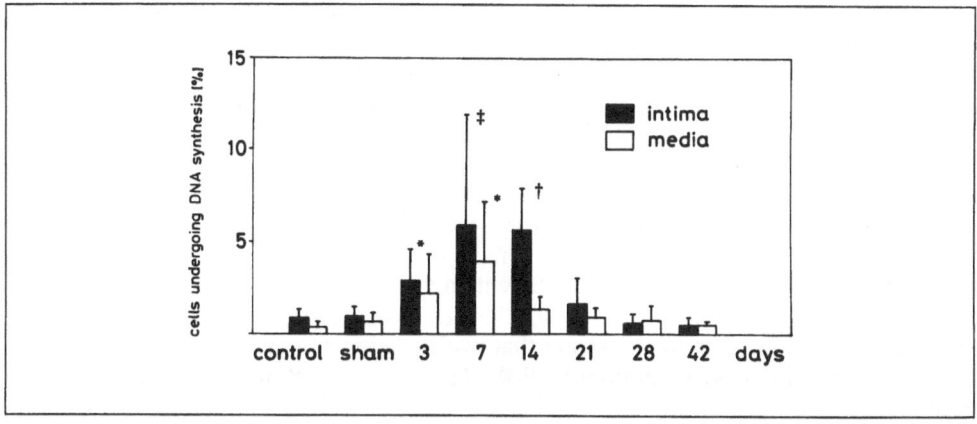

Fig. 8. Time-course of intimal and medial SMC proliferation following excimer laser ablation. The results of 36 arteries after determination of the extent of SMC undergoing DNA synthesis in both layers using bromodeoxyuridine-labeling are shown. All values are expressed in mean ±SD (*p<0.05, †p<0.01, ‡p<0.25=n. s.).

dynamic process with a peak value of DNA synthesis during the first 7 days after balloon angioplasty. The high number of proliferating cells early after dilatation results in a continuous increase of intimal cell layers. The number of SMCs undergoing DNA synthesis, however, already decreases between days 7 and 14 after angioplasty. The phenomenon of increasing cell layers during 4 weeks following angioplasty, in spite of a decreasing DNA synthesis, is explained by proliferation of a large number of cells in the early stage. The cells proliferate further at a lower level until cell division of SMC approaches baseline level between days 21 and 28 following interventional treatment. In comparison to the intimal proliferation, medial SMC presents an increase of DNA synthesis up to 21 days following angioplasty. This prolonged increase of medial SMC proliferation can be explained in part by direct arterial injury of the medial layer induced by the intervention. Additionally, substitution of previously migrated smooth muscle cells into the intimal layer might lead to this increased medial SMC proliferation during a period of 21 days. Determination of intimal and medial SMC proliferation using thymidine analogue substances following arterial balloon injury has been previously demonstrated in rats only [45, 53]. Clowes et al. [53] found maximal SMC thymidine indices in the media at 4 days, and in the intima at 7 days after balloon injury. The model of balloon denudation in normal arteries leads to activation of medial SMC with migration and proliferation into the intimal layer with a prolonged increase of proliferation in the intimal layer. Using electrical stimulation, balloon angioplasty of a pre-existing intimal plaque was performed in our experimental setting. The time-dependent reaction of SMC due to the injury induced by balloon dilatation appears to be uniform and was observed in all dilated arteries.

Experimental excimer laser angioplasty

Several in vitro studies have demonstrated that with the energy emitted from a pulsed 308 nm excimer laser precise and efficient ablation of atherosclerotic plaque with only minimal thermal injury of the adjacent tissue can be performed [28, 29, 54, 55].

In contrast to the acute mechanisms, only limited information is available about the chronic effects following excimer laser ablation in vivo [33].

The ablation of tissue in our experiments resulted in an initial decrease of intimal cell layers in the acute setting. Interestingly, complete ablation of the intima and additional ablation and scarring of the medial layer, which occurred in 12 vessels, was associated with local reduction of cell nuclei in the adjacent tissue in the majority of these arteries.

This phenomenon may be explained by local tissue necrosis, probably induced by either thermal injury or photoacoustic effects of excimer laser ablation [56]. Similar effects, described as abnormal cell nuclei with decreased uptake of stains in histological sections, were also observed following thermal laser angioplasty [57, 58].

Furthermore, our data demonstrate that proliferation of smooth muscle cells leads to a continuous increase of intimal wall thickness during 28 days after excimer laser ablation.

Histomorphological determination of intimal plaque size in sham-operated and control animals did not show statistically significant differences, suggesting that the observed effects are indeed the result of application of excimer laser energy rather than due to purely mechanical vessel-wall irritation. This is even more important since we used the identical catheter device that was employed in clinical trials in patients with coronary artery disease [32, 33].

Quantification of cells undergoing DNA synthesis revealed no significant difference between sham-operated and control animals, demonstrating that the increased SMC proliferation after excimer laser angioplasty was due to the effect of laser ablation only.

Comparison of balloon and excimer laser angioplasties

The percentage of replicating SMC after balloon and laser angioplasties was determined using bromodeoxyuridine to analyze the time-course of the DNA synthesis in the treated arterial segment. In order to minimize cytotoxic effects, BrdU labeling was limited to a time interval of 18 h before excision of the vessels.

As described above, a maximum of cells undergoing DNA synthesis in the intima was observed within the first 7 days after balloon dilatation. In contrast, the results following laser ablation demonstrate that intimal and medial SMC proliferation reaches a maximum of DNA synthesis during the first 14 days after excimer laser treatment. However, the variability in vessel-wall reaction 7 days after laser treatment was considerable, resulting in a large standard deviation in the 7 day group.

In comparison to balloon angioplasty, the proliferative response of intimal smooth muscle cells following excimer laser ablation is delayed. The maximal rate of cells entering s-phase of mitosis after excimer laser ablation appears to be reduced to approximately 50%, compared to after balloon angioplasty. However, SMC proliferation after excimer laser ablation, as well as after balloon angioplasty, resulted in a continuous increase of intimal thickening during 28 days. Thus, the absolute extent of intimal cell layers following excimer laser treatment after 28 days is comparable to the increase of intimal cell layers after balloon angioplasty. Incidence and morphology of stenosis (>50%) due to intimal SMC proliferation are also comparable in both experimental settings.

Study implications

These results strongly support the concept of intimal hyperplasia due to proliferation of SMCs of the medial and intimal layers as a uniform process following vessel wall injury [19, 44].

Our findings are also in agreement with several autopsy reports following PTCA and one post mortem report after stand-alone excimer laser angioplasty; these reports described an intimal hyperplasia in all patients, whether or not restenosis had occurred [20, 21, 59, 60]. If increased proliferation of SMC following balloon dilatation or laser ablation results in a moderate intimal hyperplasia only, or in a hemodynamic significant restenosis, may be due to activation of macrophages, platelets, expression of growth factors, and the extent of the interventional injury [8, 14, 19, 44].

Considering the high level of SMCs during the first 7, respectively, 14 days after intervention, it appears important and necessary to reduce proliferation of SMCs with antiproliferative drugs in the early stage after successful balloon angioplasty and/or excimer laser treatment.

References

1. Dotter CT, Judkins MP (1964) Transluminal treatment of arteriosclerotic obstruction. Description of a new technique and a preliminary report of its application.Circulation 30: 654–670
2. Grüntzig AR (1978) Transluminal dilatation of coronary artery stenosis. Lancet 1: 263
3. Block PC (1985) Percutaneous transluminal coronary angioplasty: role in the treatment of coronary artery disease. Circulation 72: V-161
4. Holmes DR, Vliestra RE, Smith HC, Vetrovec GW, Kent KM, Cowley MJ, Faxon DP, Grüntzig AR, Kelsey SF, Detre KM, van Raden MJ, Mock MB (1984) Restenosis after percutaneous transluminal coronary angioplasty (PTCA): A report from the PTCA Registry of the National Heart, Lung and Blood Institute. Am J Cardiol 53: 77C
5. Kaltenbach M, Kober G, Scherer D, Vallbracht C (1985) Recurrence rate after successful coronary angioplasty. Eur Heart J 6: 276–281
6. Serruys PW, Luijten HE, Beat KJ, Geuskens R, de Feyter PJ, van den Brand M, Reiber JHC, Ten Katen HJ, van Es GA, Hugenholtz PG (1988) Incidence of restenosis after successful coronary angioplasty: a time-related phenomenon: A quantitative angiographic study in 342 consecutive patients at 1, 2, 3, and 4 month. Circulation 77: 361–372
7. Pasternak RC, Baughman KL, Fallon JT, Block PC (1980) Scanning electron microscopy after transluminal angioplasty of normal canine coronary arteries. Am J Cardiol 45: 591–598
8. Wilentz JR, Sanborn TA, Haudenschild CC, Valeri CR, Ryan TJ, Faxon DP (1987) Platelet accumulation in experimental angioplasty: time course and relation to vascular injury. Circulation 75: 636–642
9. Castaneda-Zuniga WR, Formanek A, Tadavatrhy M, Vlodaver Z, Edwards JE, Zollikofer C, Amplatz K (1980) The mechanism of balloon angioplasty. Radiology 135: 565–571
10. Lyon RT, Zarins CK, Lu CT, Yang CF, Gladov S (1987) Vessel, plaque, and lumen morphology after transluminal balloon angioplasty. Quantitative study in distended human arteries. Arteriosclerosis 1987; 7: 306–314
11. Block PC, Myler RK, Sterzer S, Fallon JT (1981) Morphology after transluminal angioplasty in human beings. N Engl J Med 305: 382–385
12. Sanborn TA, Faxon DP, Haudenschild CC, Gottsman SB, Ryan TJ (1983) The mechanism of transluminal angioplasty: evidence for formation of aneurysmas in experimental atherosclerosis. Circulation 68: 1136–1140
13. McBride W, Lange RA, Hillis LD (1988) Restenosis after successful coronary angioplasty. N Engl J Med 318: 1734–1737

14. Monsen CH, Adams PC, Badimon L, Chesebro JH, Fuster V (1987) Platelet-vessel wall interactions in the development of restenosis after coronarz angioplasty. Z Kardiol 1987; 76: Suppl. 6, 23–28

15. Bernstein LR, Antoniades H, Zetter BR (1982) Migration of cultured vascular cells in response to plasma and platelet-derived factors. J Cell Sci 56: 71–82

16. Ihnatowycz IO, Winocour PD, Moore S (1981) A platelet-derived factor chemotatic for rabbit smooth muscle cells in culture. Artery 9: 316–317

17. Grotendorst GR, Seppa HEJ, Kleinman HK, Martin GR (1981) Attachment of smooth muscle cells to collagen and their migration toward plateled-derived growth factor. Proc Nat Acad Sci USA 78: 3669–3672

18. Seppa H, Grotendorst G, Seppa S, Schiffmann E, Martin G (1982) Platelet-derived growth factor is chemotactic for fibroblasts. Cell Biol Int Rep 5: 813–819

19. Ross R (1986) The pathogenesis of atherosclerosis – an update. N Engl J Med 20: 488–500

20. Essed CE, van den Brand M, Becker AE (1983) Transluminal coronary angioplasty and early restenosis. Fibrocellular occlusion after wall laceration. Br Heart J 49: 393–396

21. Austin GE, Ratliff NB, Hollmann J, Tabei S, Phillips DF (1985) Intimal proliferation of smooth muscle cells as an explanation for recurrent coronary artery stenosis after percutaneous transluminal coronary angioplasty. J Am Coll Cardiol 6: 369–375

22. Steele PM, Chesebro JH, Stanson AW, Holmes DR Jr, Dewanjee MK, Badimon L, Fuster V (1985) Balloon angioplasty: Natural history of the pathophysiological response to injury in a pig model. Circ Res 57: 105–112

23. Selzer PM, Murphy-Chutorian D, Ginsburg R, Wexler L (1985) Optimizing strategies for laser angioplasty. Invest Radiol 20: 860–866

24. Isner JM, Donaldson RF, Funai JT, Deckelbaum LI, Pandian NG, Clarke RH, Konstam MA, Salem DN, Bernstein JS (1985) Factors contributing to perforations resulting from laser coronary angioplasty. Circulation 72: II 191–199

25. Abela GS, Crea F, Smith W, Pepine CJ, Conti CR (1985) In vitro effects of argon laser radiation on blood; quantitative and morphological analysis. JACC 5: 231–237

26. Abela G, Norman S, Cohen R, Feldman R, Geiger F, Conti CR (1982) Effects of carbon dioxide, Nd-YAG and argon laser radiation on coronary atheromatous plaque. Am J Cardiol 50: 1129–1205

27. Gerrity R, Loop F, Golding L, Ehrhart L, Argenyi Z (1983) Arterial response to laser operation for removal of atherosclerotic plaques. J Thorac Cardiovasc Surg 85: 409–421

28. Lawrence PF, Dries DJ, Moatamed F, Dixon J (1984) Acute effects of argon laser on human atherosclerotic plaque. J Vasc Surg 1: 852–859

29. Isner J (1986) The paradox of thermal ablation without thermal injury. Proceedings 3rd European Laser Association; Amsterdam: Echo Med Verlag, B-609–611

30. Grundfest WS, Litvack F, Forrester JS, Goldenberg T, Swan HJC, Morgenstern L, Fishbein M, McDermid S, Rider DM, Pacala TJ, Laudenslager JB (1985) Laser ablation of human atherosclerotic plaque without adjacent tissue injury. JACC 5: 929–933

31. Srinivasan R, Leigh W (1982) Ablative photodecomposition: Action of far ultraviolet (193 nm) laser radiation on poly (ethylene terephthalate) films. J Am Chem Soc 104: 6784–6785

32. Karsch KR, Haase KK, Mauser M, Ickrath O, Voelker W, Duda S, Seipel L (1989) Percutaneous coronary excimer laser angioplasty: Initial clinical results. Lancet 2: 647–650

33. Karsch KR, Haase KK, Voelker W, Baumbach A, Mauser M, Seipel L (1990) Percutaneous coronary excimer laser angioplasty in patients with stable and unstable angina pectoris: Acute results and incidence of restenosis during 6-month follow-up. Circulation 81: 1849–1859

34. Litvack F, Grundfest W, Margolis J, Eigler N, Segalowitz J, Hestrin L, Rothbaum D, Linnemeier T, Goldenberg T, Forrester J (1989) Complications during excimer laser angioplasty are similar to those during PTCA (abstract). Circulation 80 (suppl II): II–254

35. Margolis JR, Litvack F, Grundfest W, Eigler N, Goldenberg T, Laudenslager J, Tsoi D, Wong S, Segalowitz J, Hestrin L, Rothbaum D, Linnemeier T, Helfant R, Forrester J (1980) Excimer laser coronary angioplasty: results of a multicenter study (abstract). Circulation (suppl II): II–477

36. Betz E, Schlote W (1979) Responses of vessel walls to chronically applied electrical stimuli. Basic Res Cardiol 74: 10–20

37. Betz E, Hämmerle H (1984) Arterienwandproliferate und Zellkulturen als Indikatoren für Hemmstoffe der Atherogenese. Funkt Biol Med 3: 46–55

38. Hanke H, Strohschneider T, Oberhoff M, Betz E, Karsch KR (1990) Time course of smooth

muscle cell proliferation in the intima and media of arteries following experimental angioplasty. Circ Res 67: 651–659

39. Strohschneider T, Hämmerle H, Betz E (1988) Evidence for the development in phases of stenosing processes of arteries with a method of quanifying cell-kinetic reactions of smooth muscle cells in experimentally induced intima cushions (abstract). Pflügers Arch 412 (suppl 1): 56
40. Guesdon JL, Ternyck T, Avrameas S (1979) The use of avidinbiotin interaction in immunoenzymatic techniques. J Histochem Cytochem 27: 771–776
41. Falini B, de Solas I, Halverson C, Parker JW, Taylor CR (1982) Double labelled antigen method for demonstration of intracellular antigens in paraffin-embedded tissues. J Histochem Cytochem 30: 21–26
42. Hanke H, Haase KK, Hanke S, Oberhoff M, Hassenstein S, Betz E, Karsch KR (1991) Morphological changes and smooth muscle cell proliferation following excimer laser treatment. Circulation: 83; 1380–1389
43. Sachs L (1978) Angewandte Statistik. 5. Auflage. Berlin Springer Verlag
44. Liu WM, Roubin GS, King III SB (1989) Restenosis after coronary angioplasty, potential biologic determinants and role if intimal hyperplasia. Circulation 79: 1374–1387
45. Clowes AW, Schwartz SM (1985) Significance of quiescent smooth muscle migration in the injured rat carotid artery. Circ Res 56: 139–145
46. Faxon DP, Weber VJ, Haudenschild CC, Gottsman SB, McGovern WA, Ryan TJ (1982) Acute effects of transluminal angioplasty in three experimental models of atherosclerosis. Arteriosclerosis 2: 125–133
47. Clowes AW, Reidy MA, Clowes MM (1983) Mechanisms of stenosis after arterial injury. Lab Invest 49: 208–215
48. Grünwald J, Haudenschild CC (1984) Intimal injury in vivo activates vascular smooth muscle cell migration and explant outgrowth in vitro. Arteriosclerosis 4: 183–188
49. Kling D, Holzschuh T, Betz E (1987) Temporal sequence of morphological alterations in artery walls during experimental atherogenesis: occurence of leucocytes. Res Exp Med 187: 237–250
50. Betz E, Hämmerle H, Strohschneider T (1985) Inhibition of smooth muscle cell proliferation and endothelial permeability with flunarizine in vitro and in experimental atheromas. Res Exp Med 185: 325–340
51. Ross R, Glomset JA (1976) The pathogenesis of atherosclerosis. N Engl J Med 295: 369–377
52. Geer JC, McGill HC Jr, Strong JP (1968) The fine structure of human atherosclerotic lesions. Am J Pathol 33: 263–287
53. Clowes AW, Clowes MM (1985) Kinetics of cellular proliferation after arterial injury II. Inhibition of smooth muscle growth by heparin. Lab invest 52: 611–616
54. Linker R, Srinivasan R, Wynne JJ, Alonso DR (1984) Farultraviolet laser ablation of atherosclerotic lesions. Lasers Surg Med 4: 201–206
55. Leon MB, Underhill DJ, Smith PD (1986) Excimer lasers for angioplasty: comparison of KrF and XeCl and mechanism of tissue ablation (abstract). JACC 7: 207 A
56. Cross FW, Al-Dhahir RK, Dyer PE (1988) Ablative and acoustic response of pulsed UV laser-irradiated vascular tissue in a liquid environment. J Appl Phys 64: 2194–2201
57. Prevosti LG, Leon MB, Smith PD, Dodd JT, Bonner RF, Robinowitz M, Clark RE, Virmani R (1988) Early and late healing responses of normal canine artery to excimer laser irradiation. J Thorac Cardiovasc Surg 96: 150–156
58. Macruz R, Ribeiro MP, Brum JM (1985) Laser surgery in enclosed spaces: a review. Lasers Surg Med 5: 199–218
59. Giraldo AA, Esponso OM, Meis JM (1985) Intimal hyperplasia as a cause of restenosis after percutaneous transluminal coronary angioplasty. Arch Pathol Lab Med 109: 173–175
60. Karsch KR, Haase KK, Wehrmann M, Hassenstein S, Hanke H (1991) Smooth muscle cell proliferation and restenosis after stand alone coronary excimer laser angioplasty. JACC 17: 991–994

Author's address:
Hartmut Hanke, M. D.
Department of Medicine
Division of Cardiology
Otfried-Müller-Str. 10
D-7400 Tübingen, FRG

Coronary Laser Angioplasty: Clinical Experience

H. J. Geschwind

Director, Cardiac Catheterization Laboratory and Interventional Cardiology, Professor, University of Paris XII, University Hospital Henri-Mondor, Créteil, France

Introduction

Interventional cardiology started in 1977 when Gruentzig in Zurich, Switzerland, performed the first percutaneous transluminal coronary angioplasty (PTCA). The first procedure was successful and he was able to pursue this technique. It proved to be a breakthrough in the treatment of cardiovascular disease and especially coronary disease, because, up to then, only medical treatment or surgical by-pass procedures had been proposed for patients with coronary stenosis. The advantage of the interventional cardiology procedure was a relative safety, a short hospitalization, a quick recovery, and no need for anesthesia. Thus, balloon dilatation became one of the most frequently used treatments, inducing numerous hospitals to become involved in the technology.

Improvement in the balloon catheter design, namely, lower profile, compliant or non-compliant balloons, decreased catheter shaft, smoother distal tips, and over-the-wire technology allowed more arteries (both proximal and distal), and tortuous vessels to be treated, thus extending the indications. The primary success rate became high, and the complication rate dramatically decreased as the technique improved, making dilatation both safe and effective.

However, the long-term follow-up did not generate the same enthusiasm among interventional and non-interventional cardiologists. It rapidly appeared that the restenosis rate was higher than originally anticipated. This was thought to be due to the drawbacks of the method itself that included the pushing aside of obstructing material, splitting, fracturing, and fissuring of the atheromatous plaque, and stretching the healthy side of the arterial wall. The consequences of balloon inflation included deep damage to the wall, with lesions inflicted not only to the intima, but also to the media and even occasionally to the adventitia. Obviously, catheter manipulations and wall-stretching were likely to result in endothelial denudation. This in turn could lead to platelet agregation and thrombus formation.

Recent reports [1] confirmed the hypothesis that restenosis after dilatation was due to smooth muscle cell proliferation, with intimal proliferation occurring within 6 months after the procedure. The extent of intimal proliferation was greater in lesions with evidence of medial or adventitial tears than in lesions with no or only intimal tears. A deeper vascular injury is associated with a greater intimal proliferation [2]. A greater inflation pressure results in more extensive arterial injury followed by greater smooth muscle cell proliferation. Thus, best initial results must be obtained with minimal injury to the vessel wall.

The concept of atherectomy: laser angioplasty

Taking into account these facts, it was thought from the early 1980s that ablating atheroma could result in better results than by pushing it aside. Moreover, this kind of procedure could prevent deep injury to the vessel wall from occurring. Laser energy was thought to be suitable for removal of obstructing material since a high energy level is available that can be transmitted through flexible optical fibers which can be tracked to distal vessels from a remote source of energy toward the atheromatous target [3]. There were great expectations, but deep disappointment followed. Indeed, it was rapidly realized that laser technology is extremely difficult to be applied in vessels because the laser catheter must be targeted to the lesion, wall perforation must be avoided, and precise cuts must be obtained. This was the main reason for the development of the hot-tip lasers which had not to be aimed at the obstruction since the effect was only a heat dissipation around the olive-shaped metal tip [4]. Despite this limitation, success was reported in peripheral arterial obstructions even though late reports suggested that the mechanical effect of the catheter was likely to play the major role. However, the use of thermal angioplasty was restricted to peripheral arteries where heat can be dissipated without major risk. This was not the case for the treatment of coronary lesions. Preliminary trials using this technique had a high rate of complications, including thrombus formation, acute closures, and embolization. Therefore, it was speculated that "cold lasers" (such as pulsed lasers) had a better chance to be successfully used in coronary arteries with a reasonable safety. Moreover, experimental studies conducted in the early 1980s had shown that pulsed lasers such as the ultraviolet excimer laser was able to create smooth-edged cuts with little if any thermal damage [5]. The fact that in some specimens an irregular, torn shape could be observed was not taken into account. It turned out from further experiments that this process was not necessarily artificial, but that pressure or accoustic shock waves might have been involved.

The question that is raised by these findings is still whether it is crucial or not to leave an even surface on the internal vessel lumen after laser irradiation, when in most cases a balloon dilatation is required which obviously inflicts severe damage to the endothelium, the intima, and even the outer layers of the vessel wall. Although preliminary studies have shown that thermal damage to the surrounding tissue after laser irradiation does not depend upon the wavelength, but on the repetition rate, namely the thermal relaxation time that allows the tissue to cool between each laser emission, it appears that the efficiency of infrared, pulsed dye or ultraviolet lasers is different [5]. The energy required to ablate a given volume of tissue depends on the absorption characteristics. For instance, it was shown that the ultraviolet excimer was absorbed by proteins, the dye laser was preferentially absorbed by yellow atheroma, and the infrared Nd YAG, Holmium YAG has a good absorption by water. The energy required for tissue ablation by infrared lasers was higher than that required by ultraviolet. Therefore, both the thermal damage and the pressure waves were thought to be greater with infrared than with ultraviolet lasers.

As mentioned by Isner et al. [6], the demonstration that laser light can convert atheromatous plaque into gas-phase vapors that are soluble in blood, and that such laser light can be transmitted through thin optical fibers suggested that laser could be used to recanalize totally occluded arteries. This was actually the first step in the clinical application of laser angioplasty. The field of studies was preferentially peripheral arteries such as the superficial femoral artery, because 1) it is a straight vessel in which stiff catheters can be inserted, 2) it is a "forgiving" artery since it is usually "protected" by a network of collaterals from the arteria profunda femoris, and 3) in case of perforation there is no high risk of bleeding since the artery is totally occluded and only a limited hematoma is likely to occur. The major limitation for extensive studies in this artery is the relative indication for recanalization. Indeed, it was thought that there is no strong indication for recanalizing totally occluded femoral arteries in patients who present only with mild claudication since symptoms are mild, distal flow is sufficient because of collaterals, and risk of reclosure is high, as observed from previous balloon angioplasty follow-up reports. On the other hand, it may be stated that recanalization of a totally occluded or severely stenosed artery may be indicated because of relief of symptoms and improved distal vessel flow, provided that the procedure is harmless, easy to perform, painless and performed without anesthesia, and with a short hospitalization. This is actually the case with interventional procedures such as conventional dilatation, laser angioplasty or laser-assisted balloon angioplasty.

The plan of our Unit and the laser research group was: 1) to demonstrate that laser angioplasty is a feasible technique, able to create a channel through totally occluded arteries; 2) to extend the procedures to peripheral arteries with a more sophisticated technique, and 3) to move from the easier and more forgiving field of straight and large peripheral arteries to the more difficult field of the fragile, tiny, and tortuous coronary arteries.

Laser peripheral artery angioplasty

Our first objective was achieved in 1983, 1984. After experimental studies conducted with a continuous wave neodymium yttrium aluminum garnet laser coupled to a 0.4-mm optical fiber inserted into a balloon catheter, we were able to recanalize totally occluded or severely stenosed femoro-popliteal arteries. The experimental studies showed that craters and holes could be created through both normal and atheromatous tissue with extensive thermal damage. Further studies also showed that the size and amount of debris generated by laser irradiation were small enough to avoid major distal embolization. Since these observations were in agreement with other studies, we had no concern about the clinical risk. To minimize the consequences of heat dissipation using continuous wave laser with a major thermal effect, saline was perfused during laser irradiation [7]. Moreover, to keep the optical bare fiber in the center of the arterial lumen, a centering inflated balloon was used. By doing so, our angiographic studies were able to show that recanalization could be achieved and channels created in tight stenoses beside the original channel, so that the final result showed a significant enlargement. Histologic sections of treated vessels obtained after amputation indicated that: 1) laser irradiation was able to ablate the obstruction, 2) no thrombus could be seen at the site of laser angioplasty, and 3) residual thermal effect with necrosis, coagulation, and vacuoles in the surrounding vessel wall tissue was still present 2 weeks after the procedure [8].

"Hot" and "cold" lasers

At that time, laser research groups had divergent opinions on whether heat should be used or avoided, or replaced by "cold" lasers such as pulsed lasers. On the one hand, thermal angioplasty was extensively developed and utilized with the hot-tip laser in peripheral arteries, and on the other hand, it was claimed that only pulsed lasers have the capability of ablating clacified material without heat dissipation, thrombus formation or dissection. These were the reasons why we moved from the solid-state, reliable, continuous wave Nd YAG laser to the more sophisticated and complex pulsed dye laser [9]. This particular wave length had been shown to ablate tissue with minimal if no

69

thermal effect [10]. Moreover, experimental studies had demonstrated that this particular wavelength is preferentially absorbed by atheromatous tissue [11]. Therefore, less energy could be used to ablate obstructing material so that it could possibly be maintained below the threshold for effective healthy tissue ablation. A series of 128 consecutive patients were candidates for laser recanalization because of symptoms related to ischemia of the lower extremities and total occlusion of the femoro-popliteal or the iliac artery. Since in 53 patients conventional techniques were successful in recanalizing the artery, in the remaining patients laser angioplasty was attempted using a single 0.2-mm fiber inserted into a centering balloon or a modified Van Andel catheter. In addition, the system was equipped with a diagnostic laser aimed at inducing tissue fluorescence via the same fiber [12]. Since the spectrum was different in atheromatous and healthy tissue the diagnostic computerized tool was able to activate the treatment laser only when obstructing atheroma was recognized, and to inhibit laser emission in case of normal tissue detection. We could recanalize occluded arteries in 82% of patients with the adjunct of balloon angioplasty in order to enlarge the narrow pilot hole created by the thin fiber, regardless of the occlusion length, but with a lower success rate in calcified lesions. Acute reclosures occurred and perforations could be detected, but as mentioned earlier, due to the site of a forgiving artery there were no clinical sequelae. More interestingly, the patency rate at an 18-month follow-up was 64%, which is close to that commonly reported after balloon angioplasty [13, 14]. However, given the fact that the new method of treatment was applied to severely diseased patients, these results may be considered encouraging.

Laser coronary angioplasty

Consequently, we moved to stage 3 of our program. To achieve this goal, we had to take into account the specific problems raised by the recanalization of obstructed thin, tortuous vessels, and the potential consequences of a failed procedure, namely perforation resulting in tamponade, acute ischemia resulting in myocardial infarction, and/or emergency by-pass surgery. We also kept in mind the goal of debulking the coronary artery to avoid adjunct dilatation and to leave patients on stand-alone laser therapy. For these reasons, we took advantage of the opportunity provided by new technology. The concept that was used consisted of a mechanical guidance replacing the guidance based upon tissue analysis. The mechanical guidance was derived from the commonly used guidewire in balloon angioplasty. The advantage of such a guide was the expertise in this field derived from multicenter trials conducted since the early 1980s. Interventional cardiologists involved in the preliminary trials of laser angioplasty could use almost the same method as the one they use routinely for balloon dilatation. This consisted of passing the guide wire through the lesion and advancing the new laser catheter over the guide wire [15]. The laser catheter was aimed at creating a large crater through the coronary lesion with a high trackability and flexibility. Therefore, the laser catheter was a multifiber device consisting of 14 to 40 optical fibers of 100 to 200 μm each, concentrically arranged around a central lumen for the passage of the guide wire. The overall flexibility of the fibers was anticipated to be roughly equal to that of a single fiber.

The catheter was coupled with a pulsed mid-infrared laser. The reason for such a choice was reliability, low-cost maintenance, and good transmission of high energy through the fibers. Indeed, the Holmium YAG laser used is a solid-state laser [16, 17].

70

Moreover, studies conducted in our laboratory and by others demonstrated this laser to effectively cut hard tissue such as bones [18], to be well absorbed by water, the major component of all tissues, to effectively create craters even when the distal fiber tip was kept at a distance from the target, and to provide smooth-edged cuts into tissue with a reduced thermal effect. We also were able to show that this wave length was preferentially absorbed by atheroma as compared to healthy tissue.

Several catheter designs were being used. One consisted of a tapered end aimed at mechanically pushing aside atheromatous material to be trapped for more effective laser ablation by the outer ring of fibers [19].

In this chapter, we report preliminary data on the first 53 consecutive patients with total occlusion (40%) or stenosis of the left main, the left anterior, the left circumflex, the right coronary artery or saphenous vein graft. Only tight stenoses were treated by laser angioplasty since the mean percent was 94%. Lesions were rather long, with a mean length of 6 mm. Most lesions were located on the left anterior descending artery and the right coronary artery. There were rather more complex than simple, including 45 type-B or -C, and calcified lesions [20]. It was not a randomized trial; patient selection was based on difficult lesions for dilatation, total occlusions, long calcified stenoses or ostial lesions. The primary success rate was 64%: this was defined as the laser catheter successfully crossing the lesion to obtain a reduction in stenosis of >20%. Procedure success, as defined as the ability to effectively reduce the stenosis to <40% with adjunct dilatation, was 94%. Failures were due to inability to advance the laser catheter against the lesion or to cross the obstruction during laser emission. This was due to a lack of flexibility, not at the proximal or mid-section of the catheter, but at the very distal tip where stiffness is due to the need for holding the fibers together. It also should be kept in mind that to achieve debulking, large catheters have to be used which are not easy to track through tiny tortous vessels. Since the channel diameter obtained with pulsed lasers is similar to that of the fiber diameter or the fiber bundle diameter the catheter/vessel diameter ratio should be very close to 1. This increases the tricky problem of tracking the catheter through the vessel toward the target.

Another drawback is the need for using a large guide catheter and positioning into the coronary ostium. This may impede the flow to the myocardium, create severe ischemia, and allow only for a brief laser irradiation. Moreover, the large catheter size does not allow good visualization of the coronary tree during the procedure while the laser catheter is being inserted into the guide wire and the diseased coronary artery when contrast medium is injected. Therefore, any assessment of the early result obtained by laser irradiation may be either difficult or almost impossible to obtain.

Only 18% of patients could be left on laser stand-alone therapy, whereas the remaining patients had to undergo adjunctive balloon angioplasty. The obstruction could be reduced by laser irradiation from 94% to 62% and by dilatation to 25%. Interestingly, the final result obtained after both laser and balloon angioplasty in total occlusions was very close to that observed in stenoses. In patients in whom the laser catheter failed to be passed through the occlusion success could, nevertheless, be obtained by balloon dilatation at a lower pressure inflation than during the originally failed dilatation procedure. This fact may be due to "tissue softening", a process which has not been demonstrated, but which could result from calcium redistribution and/or splitting [20]. It may facilitate the angioplasty dilatation procedure in cases of hard atheromatous calcified obstruction.

Acute occlusion (during the procedure) or early (within 24 h after the procedure) was the major complication, occuring in 19% of cases. However, in almost all cases it was possible to recanalize the artery by repeat dilatation. This fact might have been due to lack of ablation of obstructing material, thrombus formation, spasm or dissection. Dissection was observed in 28% of cases, but was significant in only 6%. The frequency of spasm induction after laser irradiation was relatively high, but could be relieved in all cases by nitrates. Rarely did it occur at the site of irradiation, and was mostly observed at a distance from the laser emission on the distal section of the treated artery.

The procedure is remarkably safe, since we observed only a single contrast medium limited extravasation that had no clinical consequence. This is due to the safe mechanical guidance over the wire. As mentioned before, acute closure or inhomogenous image within the obstruction after laser irradiation could well be due to the so-called swiss-cheese effect. The space in between the fibers was not covered by fibers, was not irradiated and, consequently, was not ablated. Therefore, some material could have been left after the procedure. This underscores the need for more densely packed fibers which are likely to reduce the "dead space". Or, there may also be a need for overlap irradiation between the fibers by optical means. Anyway, it seems that the avenue for future research would be a very flexible, thin laser catheter which is able to create large holes rather than to use a large untracktable catheter which is unable to create wide channels, but instead only creates tunnels that have to be enlarged subsequently by dilatation.

For the interventional cardiology community, a laser device is now available that is ready for routine use in the coronary arteries. Regardless of the wavelength used, infrared, dye or excimer ultraviolet, coronary obstructions can now be treated by laser irradiation and, in some cases, without adjunctive balloon dilatation. This would allow for widespread multicenter trials that could provide a short- and long-term assessment of the results obtained by laser alone. Improvement in trackability, reduction of the dead space between fibers that increases the energy density at the distal fiber tip would allow for improved results. The most exciting issue is that of the role of shock waves which were shown to be not negligible with pulsed lasers; their role in dissection or remodeling the artery is still unknown. From preliminary data concerning the late follow-up it is suggested that the rate of restenosis would be relatively high, at least not lower than that observed after dilatation. However, these cannot be considered disappointing results since laser angioplasty was primarily performed in total occlusions, long lesions, and proximal stenoses which are known to be followed by a high restenosis rate after conventional dilatation. It clearly appears that laser irradiation will be the method of choice since the laser beam can be altered to be aimed directly and exactly at the target from a remote energy source with the beam conducted through small catheters. Provided that pressure waves and thermal effects can be controlled, laser energy will be able to remove atheroma without damage to the arterial wall. This is far from being the case with dilatation, whose future may be limited because of the lesions inflicted to the vessel wall layers [21] (this has been shown to induce the restenosis process), unless a revolutionary drug can be developed that would reduce or interrupt this process.

References

1. Nobuyoshi M, Kimura T, Ohishi H, Horiuchi H, Nosaka H, Hamasaki N, Yokoi H, Koutaku K (1991) Restenosis after percutaneous transluminal coronary angioplasty: pathologic observations in 20 patients. J Am Coll Cardiol 17: 433–439
2. Ip JH, Fuster V, Badimon L, Badimon J, Taubman MB, Chesebo JH (1990) Syndromes of

accelerated atherosclerosis; role of vascular injury and smooth muscle cell proliferation. J Am Coll Cardiol 15: 1667–1687

3. Abela GS, Normann S, Cohen D, Feldman RL, Geiser EA, Conti CR (1982) Effects of carbondioxide, Nd-YAG and argon laser radiation on coronary atheromatous plaques. Am J Cardiol 5: 1199–1205

4. Sanborn TA, Cumberland DC, Greenfield AJ, Welsh CL, Guben JK (1988) Percutaneous laser thermal angioplasty: initial results and 1-year follow-up in 129 femoropopliteal lesions. Radiology 168: 121–125

5. Deckelbaum LI, Isner JM, Donaldson RF, Laliberte SM, Clarke RH, Salem DN (1986) Use of pulsed energy delivery to minimize tissue injury resulting from carbon dioxide laser irradiation of cradiovascular tissues. J Am Coll Cardiol 7: 898–908

6. Isner JM, Rosenfield K, Losordo DW (1990) Excimer laser atherectomy. Circulation 81: 2018–2021

7. Geschwind HJ, Boussignac G, Teisseire B, Benhaiem N, Bittoun R, Laurent D (1984) Conditions for effective Nd-YAG laser angioplasty. Br Heart J 52: 484–489

8. Geschwind HJ, Fabre M, Chaitman B, Lefebvre-Villardebo M, Ladouch A, Boussignac G, Blair J, Kennedy HL (1986) Histopathology after Nd-YAG laser percutaneous transluminal angioplasty of peripheral arteries. J Am Coll Cardiol 8: 1089–1095

9. Geschwind HJ, Dubois-Rande JL, Shafton E, Boussignac G, Wexman M (1989) Percutaneous pulsed laser-assisted balloon angioplasty guided by spectroscopy. Am Heart J 117: 1147–1152

10. Prince MR, Anderson RR, Deutsch TF, La Muraglia GM (1988) Pulsed laser ablation of calcified plaque. SPIE 906: 305–309

11. Prince MR, Deutsch TF, Mathews-Roth MM, Margolis R, Parrish JA, Oseroff AR (1986) Preferential light absorption in atheromas in vitro. Implication for laser angioplasty. J Clin Invest 78: 295–302

12. Richards-Kartum R, Mehta A, Hayes G, Cothren R, Kolubayev T, Kittrell C, Ratcliff NB, Kramer JR, Feld MS (1989) Spectral diagnosis of atherosclerosis using an optical fiber laser catheter. Am Heart J 118: 381–391

13. Geschwind HJ, Aptecar E, Boussignac G, Dubois-Randé JL, Zelinsky R, Poirot G, Tomaru T (1991) Results and follow-up after percutaneous pulsed laser-assisted balloon angioplasty guided by spectroscopy. Circulation 83: 787–796

14. Lee G, Mason DT (1991) Laser angioplasty: a plea for modesty in the search for a real beginning. Circulation 83: 1093–1095

15. Karsch KR, Haase KK, Voelker W, Baumbach A, Mauser M, Seipel L (1990) Percutaneous coronary excimer laser angioplasty in patients with stable and unstable angina pectoris–Acute results and incidence of restenosis and 6-month follow-up. Circulation 81: 1849–1859

16. Aretz HT, Butterly JR, Jewell ER, Setzer SE, Shapsey SM (1989) Effects of Holmium-YSGG laser irradiation on arterial tissue: preliminary results. SPIE 1067: 127–132

17. Treat MR, Trokel SL, Reynolds D, De Filippi VJ, Andrew J, Ying Liu J, Cohen MG (1988) Preliminary evaluation of a pulsed 2.15 µm laser system for fiberoptic endoscopic surgery. Lasers Surg Med 8: 322–326

18. Muss RC, Fabian RL, Sarkar R, Puliafito CA (1988) Infrared laser bone ablation. Lasers Surg Med 8: 381–391

19. Geschwind HJ, Dubois-Rande JL, Murphy-Chutorian D, Tomaru T, Zelinsky R, Loisance D (1990) Percutaneous coronary angioplasty with mid-infrared laser and a new multifiber catheter. The Lancet 336: 245–246

20. Izatt JA, Albagli D, Itzkan I, Feld MS (1990) Pulsed laser ablation of calcified tissue: physical mechanism and fundamental parameters. SPIE 1202: 133–140

21. Waller BF, Pinkerton CA, Orr CM, Slack JD, VanTassel JW, Peters T (1991) Morphological observations late (> 30 days) after clinically successful coronary balloon angioplasty. Circulation 83 (suppl I): 28-I-41

Author's address:
Herbert J. Geschwind, M. D.
Chu Henri Mondor
51, au du Marechal de Lattre de Tassigny
F-94010 Créteil

Excimer Laser Coronary Angioplasty: American Experience with the AIS System

J. R. Margolis, S. Mehta, and the AIS Registry Investigators

Cardiovascular Laboratory, South Miami Hospital, Miami, Florida

Introduction

Since Andreas Gruntzig's first reported percutaneous dilatation of coronary arteries, in 1979 (1), a plethora of devices have been developed to perform nonsurgical dilatation of occluded and stenosed coronary arteries. Besides the wide availability of vastly improved PTCA equipment, various lasers, stents, atherectomy and angioscopy devices are broadening the applicability of interventional cardiology techniques (2-7). The new modalities may also be useful in avoiding some of the drawbacks of PTCA. Pathological and angioscopic examination of coronary arteries after even uncomplicated PTCA uniformly reveals a severely disrupted intimal surface (8-10). This intimal injury, an integral component of PTCA, may lead to early closure or late restenosis. PTCA is less successfully in long or calcified lesions, chronic total occlusions, ostial disease, diffusely diseased vessels and stenosed or occluded saphenous vein grafts (11). These limitations provided an impetus to develop technologies which could open coronary arteries without major intimal damage, and could deal effectively with coronary disease states where PTCA is impossible or less effective (12). Because laser coronary angioplasty actually removes atherosclerotic plaque, there are compelling theoretical reasons why it would be superior to PTCA for the treatment of complex lesions, and for the prevention of early abrupt closure and late restenosis (13-15).

Laser angioplasty

Laser is an acronym for Light Amplification by Stimulated Emission of Radiation (16). Laser light does not occur in nature. The sharp beam of light produced by a laser is monochromatic, collimated, and coherent. The basic elements that compose a laser are the resonant cavity, the lasing medium, and the excitation mechanism. Regardless of the output wavelength, these three elements exist in all types of laser systems. Lasers are operated in either a continuous wave or gaited fashion (16-18). In the continuous wave mode, the laser oscillates constantly to provide stable power (19). Gaited or pulsed lasers incorporate a method of interrupting the laser beam to release short bursts of energy from 0.1 to 1.0 second in duration. A laser can also be pulsed by changing the method of pumping the active medium, the power, or the temporal relationship to provide higher energy output. Q-switched lasers have extremely short pulses in association with energy densities several orders of magnitude higher than other lasers, thereby providing a mechanism of rapid tissue absorption and recovery.

75

Continuous vs pulsed lasers

Pulsed lasers, in comparison to continuous lasers, affect target tissue without minimal heat dispersion or damage to surrounding structures (20). Depth of ablation varies directly with the number of pulses, and inversely with tissue density, with incision width remaining constant (21). At very high energy densities pulsed laser energy may create acoustic damage. Excimer laser energy at densities appropriate for ablation of atherosclerotic tissue and calcium does not cause clinically significant acoustic damage. Continuous wave lasers ablate via a thermal mechanism, the physical basis of which relies on the transformation of photon energy to heat. This creates tissue temperatures of several hundred degrees celsius, resulting in vaporization of contacted tissue. Microscopic and histological appearance of such tissue demonstrates a zone of concentric carbonization and coagulation necrosis caused by the denaturization of proteins (22). Continuous wave lasers in most common clinical use include Argon, ND:YAG, and CO_2.

Precise, non-thermal ablation without damage to surrounding tissue makes pulsed excimer laser energy superior to continuous wave energy for coronary angioplasty (23, 24). Histological appearance of the pulsed excimer ablated tissue differs remarkably from the thermal effect of continuous wave lasers. Tissue margins are extremely smooth, and there is neither carbonization nor coagulation necrosis (25–28). Injury of surrounding tissue is avoided, because pulsed excimer lasers ablate by non-thermal disruption of peptide bonds, resulting in photoablative decomposition. Non-thermal ablation results in a markedly diminished incidence of vascular spasm. The resultant smooth vascular surface is less thrombogenic with less disruption of intimal integrity. This improves the immediate and long term results of laser coronary angioplasty (29).

The excimer laser

The term excimer is an acronym for excited dimer. When certain gas mixtures are excited with high voltage electrical energy, a molecule is temporarily created. This excited molecule ceases to exist once the excitation process is removed. The Advanced Interventional System, Inc. (AIS) laser uses a mixture of xenon and hydrogen chloride, which generates a beam of ultraviolet light at 308 nanometers. When high voltage is discharged through this mixture, it strips off one electron from xenon (Xe) giving it a positive charge. These positive Xe^+ ions are attracted to the negatively charged chloride Cl^- ions, and combine to form the excited molecule Xenon Chloride* (XeCl*). Some of these molecules spontaneously emit a photon of light and separate thereafter into Xenon and chloride. As the photons travel through the excited gas mixture they strike other XeCl* molecules, and stimulate them to break apart and emit other photons which are identical in color and phase to the first photon. This chain reaction continues to cascade down the laser until the photons bounce off one of the mirrors that are aligned at either end of the resonant cavity. The resonant cavity is bound by a highly reflective mirror at the rear and a partially reflective mirror at the front. The lasing gas is suspended between these two mirrors, which are used to amplify the laser beam. As the photons oscillate in the resonant cavity, a small portion of the beam is permitted to escape through the partial mirror, and this becomes the usable laser beam.

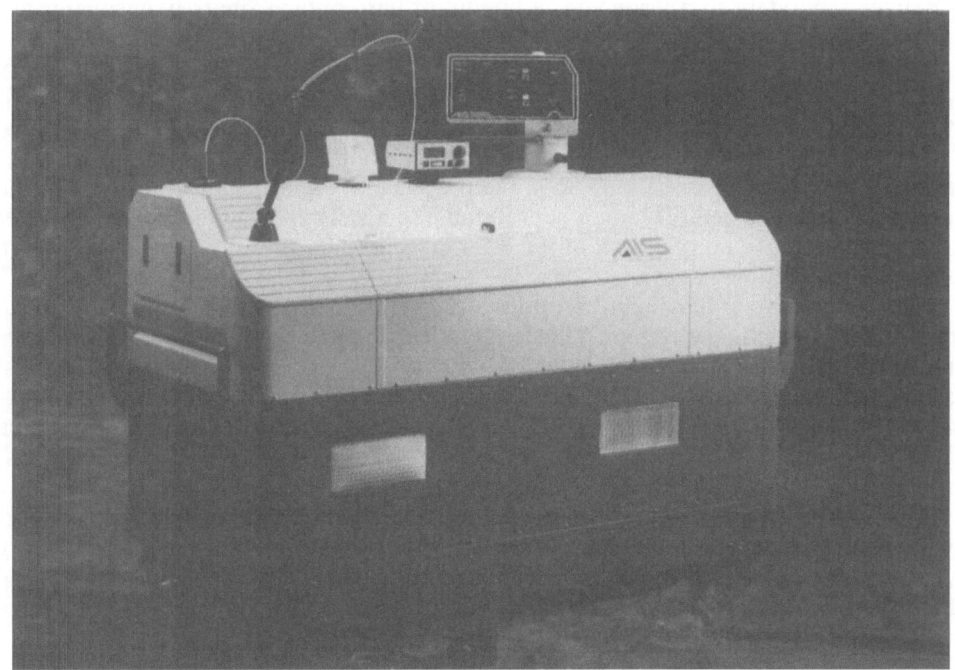

Fig. 1. Dymer Beam 200+ for coronary laser angioplasty.

The AIS equipment

The commonly used AIS Dymer Beam 200+ (Fig. 1) is an extremely long-pulse, XeCl Excimer laser, operating in the ultraviolet spectrum of 308 nm. This delivers approximately 200 mJ of energy with a pulse width in excess of 200 nanoseconds. All of the basic components are housed in one frame, which does not require any facility modifications (30). The Dymer 200+ incorporates all operator controls into a functional panel that can be viewed from any position. The control section allows the operator to select one of six pulse repetition rates, ranging from 5 hz to 30 hz in 5 hz increments. Output energy can be monitored while the catheter is inserted into the specifically designed energy meter housing. Mechanical gimbels provide precise control of the amount of energy delivered to the distal end of the fiberoptic catheter. Gas exchanges are made simple by a self-contained gas storage and administration system.

Problems relating to the design of laser coronary angioplasty systems are outlined in Table 1. The AIS system overcomes many of these problems. Because excessive peak power will destroy optical fibers, it is desirable to deliver energy over relatively long pulse widths (31, 32). Optical fibers are intrinsically inflexible: the larger the diameter, the less flexible the fiber. Very thin fibers (100 µm or less) are sufficiently flexible to track virtually anywhere within the coronary arterial tree. However, such small fibers do not remove enough material to effectively ablate coronary artery stenoses. By bundling multiple thin fibers it is possible to obtain reasonably large ablative surfaces while maintaining flexibility. Early experiments with bare optical fibers usually resulted in vessel perforation. Since bare-tipped fiberoptics are difficult to deliver accurately to a large site, a bundle of bare optical fibers is unsuitable for the delivery of energy within coronary arteries.

Table 2 lists some of the elements necessary for developing a fiberoptic delivery system for laser coronary angioplasty. By arranging the fiberoptic bundle around a central lumen, it is possible to increase total ablative area while providing room for a coaxial guide wire. An over-the-wire system helps maintain coaxial orientation of laser catheters within target vessels, even in the presence of significant tortuosity. For the purpose of safety, a central lumen is preferable to a rail-type catheter since the latter may allow eccentric margination of the laser cutting surface (although the rail design may offer other advantages).

The combination of bundled fiberoptics and a central lumen creates significant dead space within the delivery system. This leads to inefficient laser abalation, while accentuating mechanical effects. Small catheters with densely packed fibers and small central lumens are more efficient cutting tools, but cut relatively small holes. Because maximum catheter tip energy density (fluence) is inversely related to cross-sectional area when laser output is constant, smaller catheters can be used with higher fluences, thereby facilitating ablation of calcium.

In order to enhance delivery through angioplasty guiding catheters and protect coronary arteries from the relatively sharp tips of fiberoptic bundles, modern delivery systems include plastic (vinyl or polyethylene) shells which are coated with lubricating chemicals. It is important that the shell be thin enough that it does not create excessive

Table 1. Problems relating to design of laser coronary angioplasty system.

Fundamental problems
Laser-tissue interactions
Wave length
Delivery system
  –Catheter based
  –Flexible

Problems with fiberoptic systems
Wave length
Energy tolerance
Flexibility
Dead space

Safety considerations
front firing over short distance
Over the wire
Reasonable catheter/artery ratio

Table 2. Requirements for laser energy delivery system.

Flexible fiberoptic bundle
Central lumen
Acceptable amount of dead space
Plastic shell
Coupler
Acceptable size
Reliability

dead space around the lasers bundle cutting tip. The entire delivery package must be small enough to pass through a standard PTCA guiding catheter.

Fiberoptic catheter delivery systems need to be coupled to lasers in such a way that fiber bundles are protected from excessive energy peaks, but with minimum energy loss. Systems must be strong enough to deliver uniform energy during multiple passes and catheter exchanges.

In developing a system for laser coronary angioplasty, safety should be a primary consideration. In the periphery, angioplasty complications are generally manageable and are rarely life threatening. Similar complications in coronary arteries, especially perforations, may be fatal. Safety can be designed into a coronary laser system. Unfortunately, many features that make a system safe compromise its ability to perform better. A front-firing system, especially one that ablates only a short distance in front of the catheter, is much less likely to perforate than is a system which is focused through a lens at the tip (33). However, ablative area of the front firing system is limited to the cross-sectional area of the catheter tip. By following a central guide wire, a laser catheter is unlikely to deviate greatly from coaxial orientation, but such a system is limited to treatment of coronary artery lesions that can be crossed with a guide wire. When the ablative diameter of the laser catheter approaches the diameter of the normal artery, the risk of perforation is increased. At ratios close to 1:1, any lumen eccentricity or tortuosity will result in lateral deviation of the ablative surface. With catheter to vessel ratios of less than 0.67, the risk of perforation is small, but residual stenosis of more than 30% must be expected.

The coronary laser angioplasty system developed by Advanced Interventional Systems (AIS), Irvine, California, USA, couples a 308 nm excimer laser to multifiber over-the-wire catheters of 1.3, 1.6, 2.0, 2.2, and 2.4 mm diameters. Laser output is 200–300 mJ with energy fluences at the catheter tip of 35–65 mJ/mm^2. Pulse rate is variable between 5 and 30 Hz. The laser is unique in its long pulse width (>200 ns). This permits the delivery of higher energies through smaller fibers than is possible with excimer lasers systems which employ shorter pulse widths (34). The original 1.6 mm laser catheter contains a fiberoptic bundle of 12 100-μm fibers, arrayed around a central lumen which accommodates a 0.018 inch guide wire (Fig. 2). By expansion of the 100-μm fibers to 200 μm at the tip, it has been possible to maintain a small shaft size and maximum flexibility without sacrificing cutting surface (21). Newer catheter designs employ up to 200 50-μm fibers, densely packed around a central core. The laser catheters are front-firing, and ablate only a distance of 100 μm distal to their tips. Thus, ablation only takes place when the catheter is in contact with the tissue, and the expected ablation rate is relatively slow (approximately 1–2 mm/s at 20 Hz). Because the laser only ablates on contact, lasing can take place in a blood field. Absorption of laser energy by blood offers a further margin of safety.

Techniques of performing excimer laser coronary angioplasty

Emphasis is placed on proper case selection (35, 36). This primarily involves selecting lesions of complex morphology, lesions where attempted PTCA has previously failed, or restenosis lesions. Complex lesions include long, diffuse and/or calcified lesions, ostial disease, and chronic total occlusions (37–42). The system is also effective for ablation of saphenous vein graft stenoses (43–45). ELCA is generally avoided for first dilatation of stenosed coronary arteries which demonstrate a simple angiographic mor-

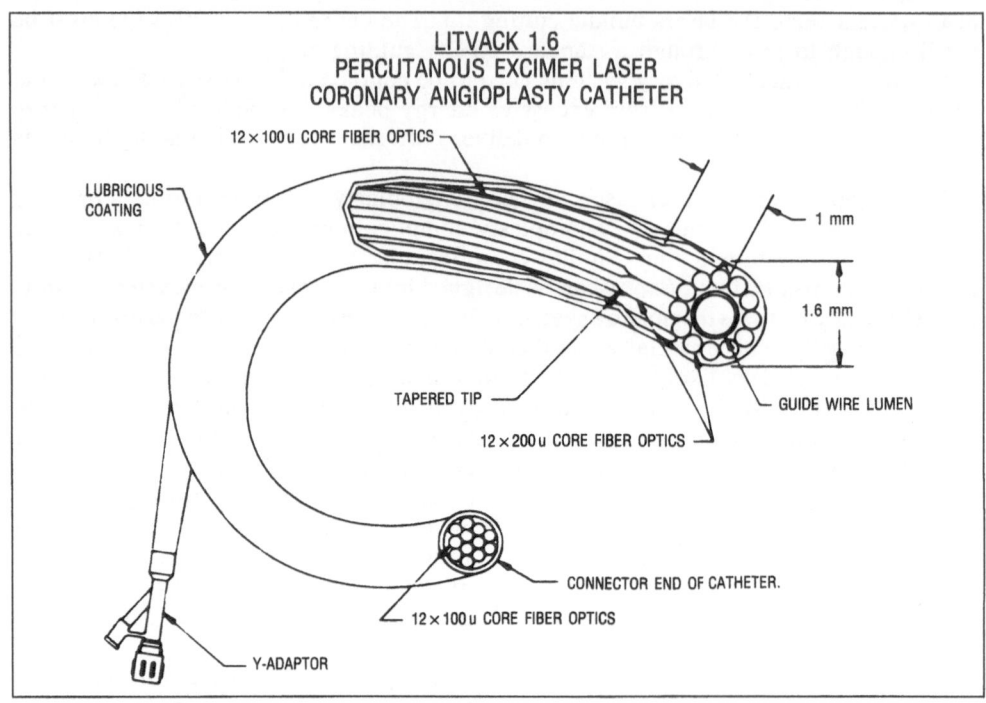

Fig. 2. Cross-section of a 1.6-mm laser catheter used for excimer laser coronary angioplasty.

phology, since such lesions are so easily done with balloon catheters. Paradoxically, hard lesions laze more easily than soft ones (46). The harder lesions resist passage of the laser catheter and thereby assure the slow catheter movement necessary for complete ablation. Tortuosity proximal to a lesion presents a greater risk of perforation, and is to be avoided (46). Tortuosity within lesions is less threatening. Lesions with tortuosity immediately distal are better suited to ELCA than PTCA, since it is necessary to laze only up to the point of tortuosity, not beyond. ELCA is effective in the treatment of unstable angina (46), but has not been used in patients with acute myocardial infarction (47). Although some studies have suggested lower restenosis rates with stand alone ELCA (48), present consensus revolves around obtaining the most optimal result, even if adjunctive balloon angioplasty is required.

ELCA patients are treated according to a protocol identical to that for standard balloon angioplasty (Table 3). Aspirin, heparin, and calcium channel blockers are used. Activated clotting times (ACT) are used to monitor heparin dosage, and are maintained between 300 and 400 s.

Large lumen PTCA guiding catheters of 8, 9, or 10 French are employed (Table 4). The 8F size suffices for 1.3 and 1.6 mm laser catheters; 9F for the 2.0 and 2.2 mm catheters; and 10F for the 2.4 mm one. Guiding catheters are selected to provide strong back-up support. This ensures that the laser continuously remains in close contact with the lesion. Excessive back-up should be avoided, since this may force the laser catheter through the lesion before lasing is complete. Generally, JL guiding catheters are used for LAD lesions; AL catheters for circumflex lesions; hockey stick, AL or

AR catheters for the RCA; and hockey stick or AR guiders for saphenous vein grafts. Coaxial orientation of the guider is important.

ELCA catheters track well over conventional 0.018-inch and 0.016-inch PTCA quidewires. A special ELCA wire, the high-torque floppy standard wire (Advanced Cardiovascular Systems, Santa Clara, California, USA) provides a better platform for catheter tracking and prevents wobbling of the catheter during ablation. This wire has

Table 3. Techniques of excimer laser coronary angioplasty.

Pre-treatment

Aspirin
calcium channel blocker
Heparin (for unstable angina)
Surgical standby indications similar to those for PTCA
Informed consent

Post-procedure

Intensive-care monitoring as for PTCA with heparinization, intravenous nitroglycerine, aspirin.
Discontinue sheats on the following morning.
Ambulate 6–8 h post sheath removal.
Discharge home that evening.
Follow-up (thallium) treadmill testing at 1 week, 3 months, and 6 months post angioplasty.

Table 4. Techniques of excimer laser coronary angioplasty.

Laser	Guiding catheter		Guide wire	Adjunctive PTCA
	Equipment			
308 nm XeCl excimer	**Size**		0.018″	Over-the-wire conventional or rapid exchange balloon catheters. P. E. material sizing as for PTCA.
Output: 200–300 mJ	8F	1.3 mm 1.6 mm	300 cm High-torque floppy with extra support exchange wire	
Tip energy: 35–60 mJ	9F	2.0 mm		
Pulse rate: 5–50 Hz	10F	2.2 mm 2.4 mm	**For simple cases:** 0.018″	
Multifiber over-the-wire laser probes: 1.3, 1.6, 2.0, 2.2, 2.4 mm dia.	**Properties** Wide lumen good back-up support ability to deep-throat		extendable wire which may be docked	
Channel size: (Expect 2/3 of nominal vessel size) ≥ 0.8 mm (1.3 mm cath) ≥ 2.0 mm (1.6 mm cath) ≥ 1.5 mm (2.0 mm cath) ≥ 1.8 mm (2.2 mm cath) ≥ 2.0 mm (2.4 mm cath)	**Guiding cath selection** LAD: JL LCX: AL RCA: AL, Hockey Stick SVG: Hockey Stick, AR			

Other factors:
1) Biplane cineangiography for LAD, LCX, SVG. Single plane suffices for RCA.
2) DSA significantly facilitates the procedure.
3) Maintain ACT between 350–400 s.
4) Continous PA monitoring for subtle hemodynamic changes.

the stiffer shaft of a high torque standard wire combined with the floppy tip of a high torque floppy wire. Conventional high torque intermediate and high torque standard 0.018-inch wires are used for lesions that cannot be crossed with floppy wires, and primarily for chronic total occlusions. In simple cases, a laser exchange wire is used. In more complex cases, the lesion is crossed with a conventional length wire, which is subsequently extended for introduction of the laser catheter.

Lesions are crossed using a bare wire technique (49). This allows easy steering and excellent visualization from quiding catheter injections. Injections of contrast around the laser catheter should be avoided. Visualization is usually poor, and there is in vitro evidence that lasing in the presence of contrast agents produces toxic by-products (50).

ELCA procedure

Because lasing occurs at a rate of only 1–2 mm/s, it is necessary to move the laser catheter very slowly. The usual technique is to bring the catheter up to the lesion, where there will be resistance to advancement; then withdraw the catheter approximately 5 mm; and then advance slowly with the laser turned on. Lasing is performed in pulse trains of 2–4 s. Longer pulse trains may lead to build-up of gaseous material, which may promote dissection at the angioplasty site (51). If the laser catheter does not move forward at the expected rate of lasing, additional pressure may lead to dissection and/or perforation.

The initial ELCA protocol called for two or three routine passes of the laser probe across each lesion. Subsequent experience has shown that multiple passes result in greater rate of complications, especially dissection and perforation, without additional benefit. The present protocol calls for a single pass after which the laser catheter is removed, a contrast injection is made over the bare wire, and the result evaluated by digital subtraction angiography. If the result is judged inadequate, the laser catheter is reintroduced only if it is felt that the lesion was not crossed completely during the initial pass. Otherwise, the original laser catheter is exchanged for a larger size laser catheter and/or a balloon. Since the laser catheter can be expected to produce a hole no larger than its nominal size, there is no rationale for multiple passes. Exceptions of this rule are orifice lesions in native arteries and saphenous vein grafts. In these cases, it is possible to create a larger hole by adjusting guiding catheter position during subsequent passes, and thereby redirecting the laser catheter. This maneuver must be performed cautiously, since it may lead to perforation. Severe lesions in large arteries are usually treated with a smaller laser catheter followed by a larger one. Since the larger diameter catheters are intentionally contructed with a large donut of central dead space, pre-ablation with a smaller catheter is essential. Usual combinations are 1.3 mm followed by 2.0 mm and 1.6 mm followed by 2.2 mm.

Although coronary artery spasm may occur, it is easily relieved by intracoronary nitroglycerin. Spasm is prevented by pretreatment of all patients with calcium channel blocking drugs and continuous infusion of intravenous nitroglycerin, and by careful lasing technique.

The presence of transluminal haziness, significant dissection, or a large residual stenosis warrant the use of adjunctive balloon angioplasty (PTCA). Catheter exchange is facilitated by use of a rapid exchange balloon system, but conventional over-the-wire balloons are satisfactory. Balloon profile is generally not a problem, since the post ELCA lumen easily admits even high profile catheters.

Post-ELCA care is identical to that after conventional PTCA. Caveats of a successful ELCA procedure include proper case selection, optimal sizing of the laser catheter, and careful attention to laser technique.

ELCA registry

The Excimer Laser Coronary Angioplasty Registry was formed to determine the feasibility of ELCA as an alternative or adjunct to PTCA (52). Initial efforts have been directed towards testing the safety and efficacy of early generation equipment, developing and perfecting clinical technique, and improving catheter and laser delivery systems. Long-term goals are to study the effect of ELCA on restenosis, and modify equipment and techniques to obtain the best long term results. Since both the equipment and techniques are continually evolving, and meaningful data on long term efficacy requires at least 1000 patients with follow-up angiography, it will be several years before the final goal of ELCA is reached.

The ELCA registry study population

The ELCA registry collects data from all 15 American institutions investigating the AIS Excimer system (Table 5). Through August, 1990, data was available on 1519 lesions in 1284 patients. The demographic profile of the registry cohort is similar to that of a standard balloon angioplasty population. Most patients were severely symptomatic: two-thirds were in Canadian Cardiovascular Society functional classes III or IV (Fig. 3). Seventy-seven percent were men with a mean age of 62 ± 10 years. Twenty-six percent of patients previously had coronary artery bypass surgery, and 36% had had previous PTCA. Vessels approached were also distributed in a manner similar to that of a standard balloon angioplasty population (Fig. 4). Sixteen percent of lesions were in the left circumflex system. The type of vessel treated distinguishes ELCA from

Table 5. ELCA follow up registry.

Participating centers	
USA	
Cedars-Sinai Med Ctr	F Litvack/N Eigler
South Miami Hospital	J Margolis/D Krauthamer
St Vincent's, Indianapolis	D Rothbaum/T Linnemeier
Emory University Hospital	S King/J Douglas
Mayo Clinic, Rochester	J Bresnahan/D Reeder
Georgetown University Hospital	K Kent/L Satler
Washington Hospital Center	M Leon/G Pichard
Goleta Valley Hosp, S Barbara	J Vogel
Methodist Hospital, Houston	W Spencer/A Raizner
Hoag Hospital, Newport Beach	R Haskell/P McNally
Philadelphia Heart Institute	W Untereker
St. Luke's Hospital, Phoenix	M Vawter
St. Luke's Hospital, Milwaukee	F Gummins/G Doros
Mercy Hospital, Pittsburgh	V Krishnaswami
Shands Hospital, Gainesville	G Abela/J Hill

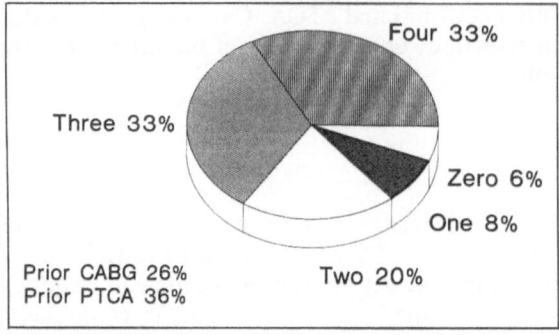

Fig. 3. ELCA registry, CCS functional class.

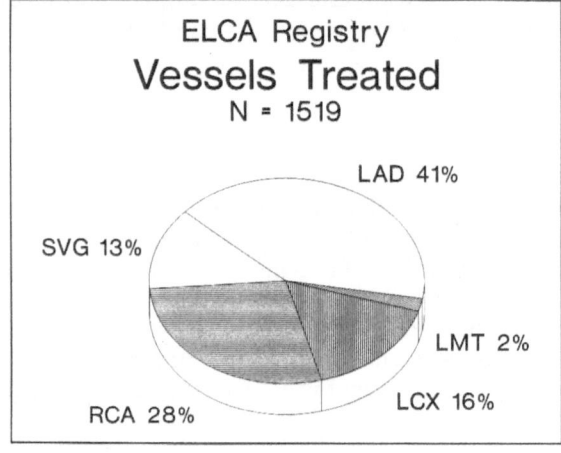

Fig. 4. ELCA registry, vessels treated.

other second generation interventional devices in that the ELCA system is capable of treating lesions in the middle and distal segments of all the coronary arteries and their branches. Thirteen percent of lesions were located in saphenous vein grafts. Ninety-one percent were stenoses; 9% were occlusions, mostly chronic total occlusions (Fig. 5). More than half of the lesions were longer than 10 mm; 21% were longer than 20 mm (Fig. 6).

The AIS system employs a 308 nm Xenon-Chloride Excimer Laser with an output of 200–300 mJ and pulse width of 200–250 ns. For the data herein reported, repetition rates of 20 Hz and catheter tip energies of 35–65 mJ/mm^2 were employed. Laser catheters of 1.3 mm (13%), 1.6 mm (64%), and 2.0 mm (24%) were used.

Results

Since the ELCA catheter produces a lumen only as large as its nominal size, a successful procedure must be defined on the basis of what can be expected. The ELCA Registry defines an acute laser success as a more than 20% reduction in stenosis diameter and

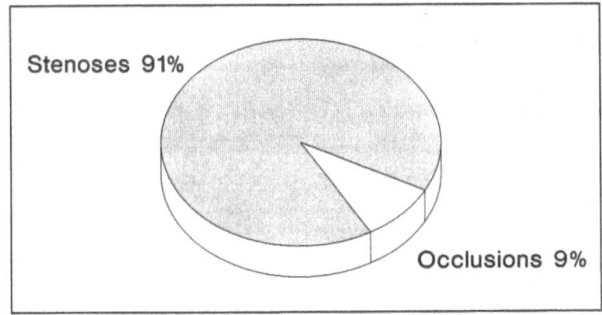

Fig. 5. ELCA registry, lesions treated.

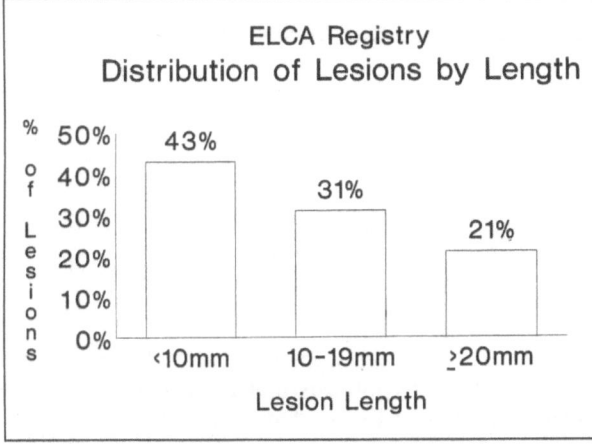

Fig. 6. ELCA registry, distribution of lesions by length.

the creation of a channel diameter by laser alone of more than 0.8 mm with a 1.3 mm catheter, more than 1.0 mm with a 1.6 mm catheter, and more than 1.5 mm with a 2.0 mm catheter. Procedure success is defined as a final diameter stenosis of less than 50% at the end of the procedure, whether or not adjunctive balloon angioplasty is performed. On the basis of these definitions, laser success was achieved in 81% of lesions, procedure success was achieved in 94%. Lesion length did not affect acute success rates (Fig. 7). Successful procedures were accomplished in 93% of lesions less than 10 mm, 96% of lesions between 10 and 19 mm, and 92% of lesions longer than 20 mm. Similarly, success rates were not affected by lesion location. Success rate for stenoses was 94%, for occlusions 91%. This is a much higher success rate than that normally associated with angioplasty of chronic total occlusions.

On the basis of caliper measurements made by individual investigators, mean diameter stenosis was reduced from 86% stenosis at baseline, to 47% post-laser, to 25% following adjunctive balloon angioplasty (Fig. 8). Quantitative coronary arteriography on a subset of these patients was in essential agreement with the caliper measurements. Using the more meaningful measurement of minimal luminal diameter, mean stenosis was increased from 0.5 mm pre-ELCA to 1.6 mm post-ELCA, to 2.1 mm

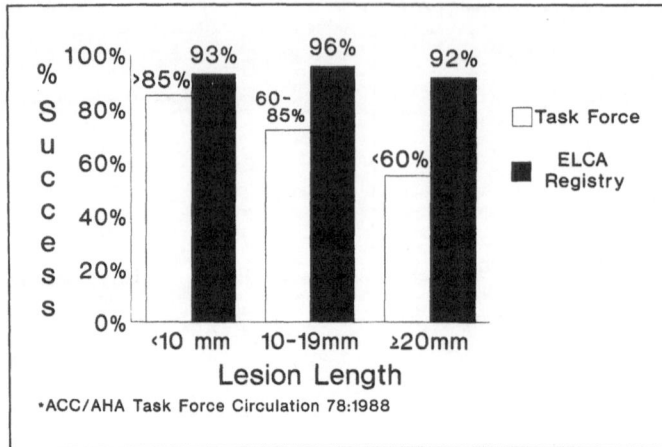

Fig. 7. Success by lesion length (ACC/AHA task force vs. ELCA registry).

BASELINE	86% ± 12%
POST ELCA	47% ± 23%
FINAL RESULT	25% ± 18%

Fig. 8. ELCA registry, stenosis severity.

post-PTCA. A 1.6 mm catheter was used for all the lesions subjected to quantitative coronary arteriography. These data support the hypothesis that the procedure works by ablation of atherosclerotic material rather than by the Dotter effect.

Although less than 50% diameter stenosis was achieved by laser alone in nearly 75% of cases, in a substantial number of these patients adjunctive balloon angioplasty was performed in an attempt to achieve the most optimal result.

The complication profile in the ELCA Registry is not dissimilar from that of a conventional balloon angioplasty population. Dissections occurred in 12% of patients, but most were clinically insignificant. Perforation occurred in 1.6% of cases (Table 6). In about half of these, the perforation lead to serious clinical sequelae requiring emergency surgery. There were no deaths due to perforation. Acute occlusion occurred in 6.5% of patients, but only 3.5% required emergency surgery. In-hospital mortality was 0.4%. Comparison of complications in the ELCA Registry vs those reported in the 1985–1986 NIH Registry demonstrates a lower incidence of non-fatal myocardial infarction, bypass surgery, and deaths in the ELCA population (Fig. 9).

Table 6. ELCA registry anatomical complications N = 1284.

Dissection	12.1%
Embolism	0.8%
Acute occlusion	6.5%
Perforation	1.6%
Spasm	1.6%
Aneurysm	0.5%

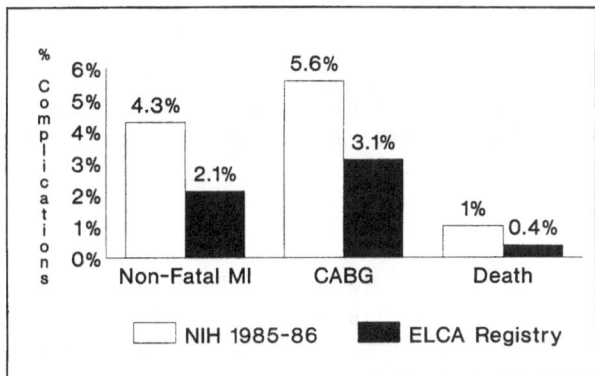

Fig. 9. Clinical complications (NIH registry vs. ELCA).

Follow-up

279 patients have been followed for 6 months; 60% of these have had repeat coronary angiography. Clinical events include death in 0.8%, myocardial infarction in 2.3%, coronary artery bypass grafting in 8.5%, and a repeat interventional procedure in 10%. The 6-month angiographic restenosis rate is 42% with a clinical restenosis rate of 17%.

South Miami Hospital ELCA series

Since South Miami Hospital (SMH) data represents approximately 25% of the entire ELCA Registry series, a closer look at these data is relevant. Through August, 1990, 279 patients had ELCA of 309 lesions. The demographic and symptom profiles of the South Miami Hospital patients are similar to those of the entire Registry series. South Miami Hospital patients had a larger proportion of left circumflex stenoses. Nearly 20% of the lesions treated with ELCA at SMH were total occlusions. Sixty percent of the lesions were in the middle and distal segments. Long lesions comprised 58% of the SMH series. For the 309 lesions, laser success was achieved in 79%, and procedure success in 92%. For the 72 total occlusions, laser success was achieved in 78%, procedure success in 96%. This means that if it is possible to cross a total occlusion with a guidewire (no matter how old or how long the lesion is) a successful result can almost always be obtained using a combination of laser and balloons (53). Although a less than 50% diameter stenosis was achieved with laser alone in 65% of lesions, 50% of lesions had adjunctive balloon angioplasty. Only 37% of the lesions were treated with laser alone (Table 7). Use of the larger 2.0 mm catheter has not significantly af-

Table 7. South Miami Hospital ELCA series stand-alone results N=309.

Stand-alone laser (50% after laser)	202 (65%)
true stand-alone*	113 (37%)

* 50% after laser and no adjunctive balloon angioplasty.

87

fected the stand-alone rate. Mean stenosis severity was reduced from 87% at baseline to 50% post ELCA, and to 27% following adjunctive balloon angioplasty.

The complication profile of the South Miami Hospital series was somewhat better than that of the entire ELCA cohort. There were two instances of perforation (0.6%); emergency surgery rate was less than 1.0% and there was one death (0.4%) (Table 8).

Future perspectives

It is evident from the initial experience of the ELCA Registry that Excimer Laser Coronary Angioplasty can be performed safely, with no more risk than that of conventional PTCA (54). With the advent of larger diameter catheters it can serve as an alternative to PTCA. Lesions that are unfavorable for PTCA: long, diffuse, and calcified stenoses, chronic total occlusions, and ostial lesions may be ideal for ELCA. Although initial restenosis data does not suggest any advantage for ELCA, improvements in equipment and technique may be helpful in this regard. ELCA should at least improve that component of restenosis that is due to inadequate angioplasty.

ELCA technology is in its early development stage, possibly equivalent to the status of PTCA, in 1980. It is reasonable to expect continuing improvements in both the laser hardware and the catheter delivery systems. Possible future developments are listed in Table 9. Even if ELCA fails to favorably affect restenosis, it should find a permanent place in interventional cardiology. Safety and efficacy of the technique are virtually proven. Even in its relatively primitive state, ELCA has been successful in treating lesions that cannot be dilated with conventional PTCA. With the promised improvements, ELCA will be applicable to a larger number of cases. It appears unlikely that ELCA will ever replace conventional PTCA, but rather it will expand the indications for, and improve the results of angioplasty procedures.

Table 8. South Miami Hospital ELCA series stand complications N=227.

Nontransluminal infraction	4 (1.8%)
Q-wave infarction*	2 (0.9%)
Surgery*	2 (0.9%)
death	1 (0.4%)

* Same patients

Table 9. Possible future developments in excimer laser coronary angioplasty.

Catheter delivery systems
Large-diameter catheters
Improved trackability of standard catheters
Laser wires for lesions not crossable with guidewire
Rail-type catheters
Side-cutting catheters

Laser systems
Smaller lasers
Microprocessor controls
Different laser sources

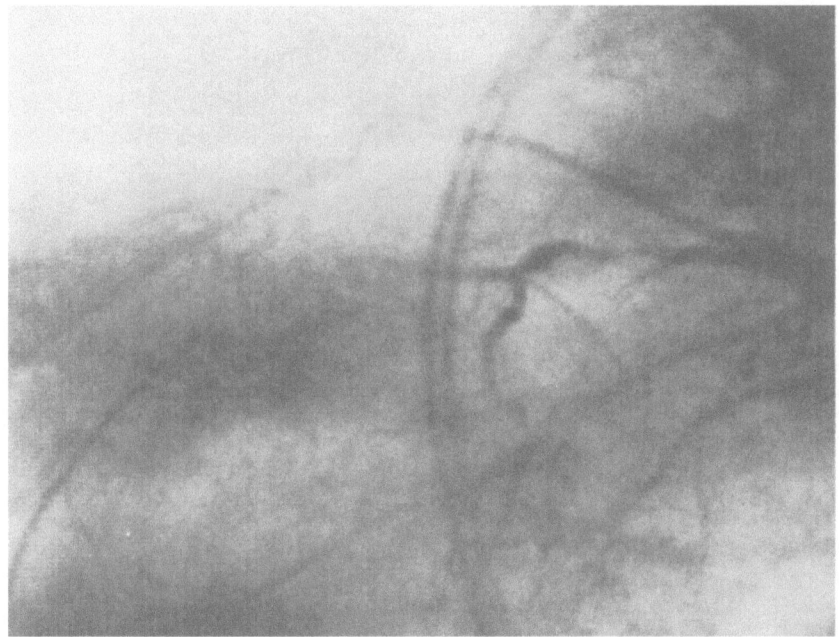

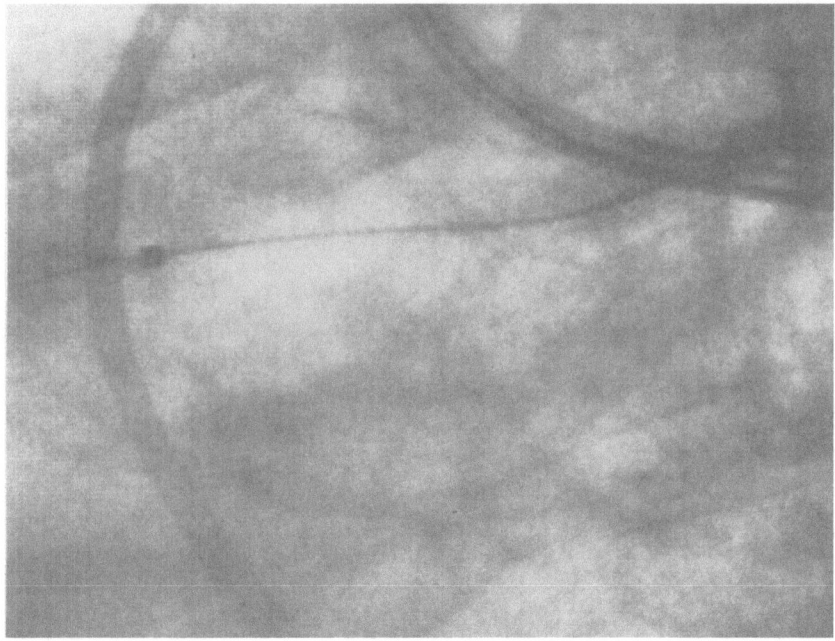

Figs. 10 a–d. 58-year-old patient with anterior wall MI 5 months prior with large antero-septal wall thallium defect: a) lateral projection revealing diffuse LAD disease; b) 1.6-mm laser across the lesion; c) immediately post-ELCA followed by adjunctive PTCA; d) 6-months post-ELCA.

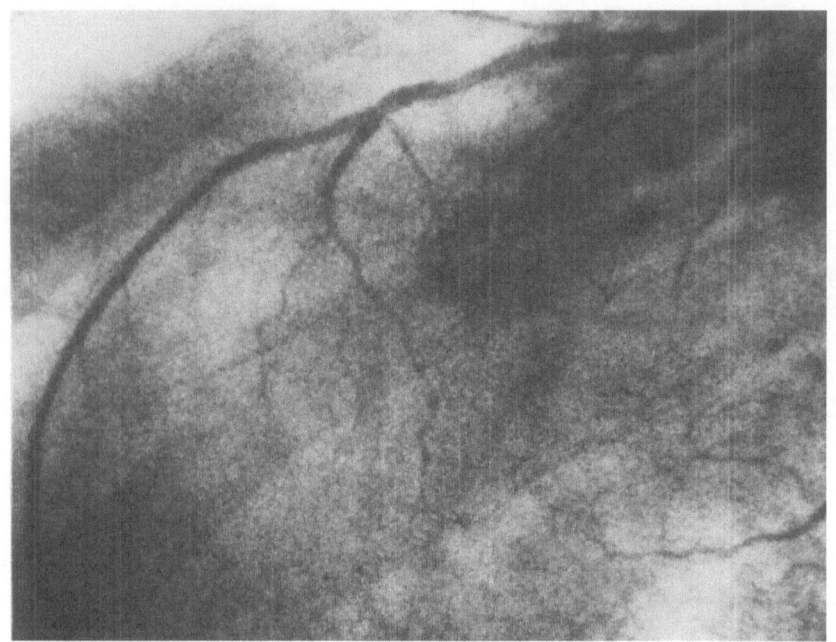

Fig. 10c.

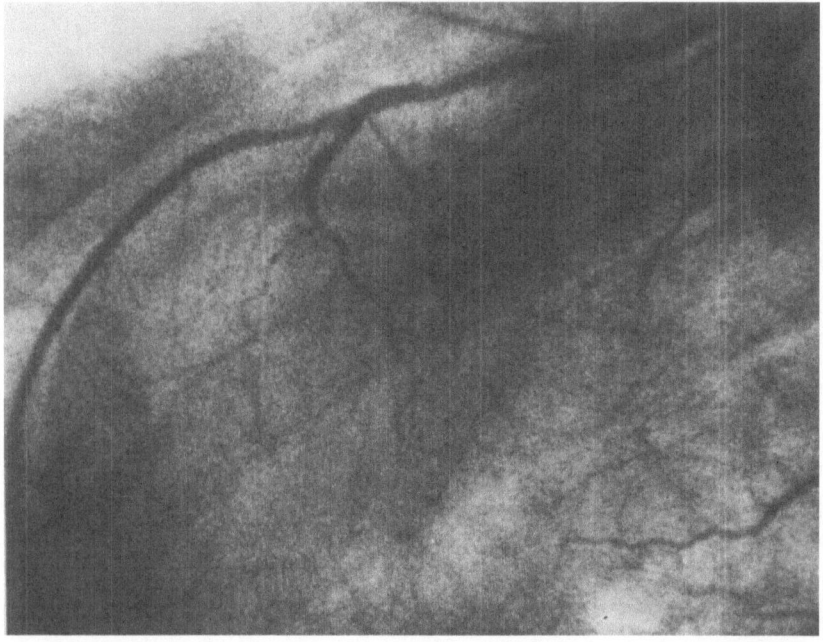

Fig. 10d.

90

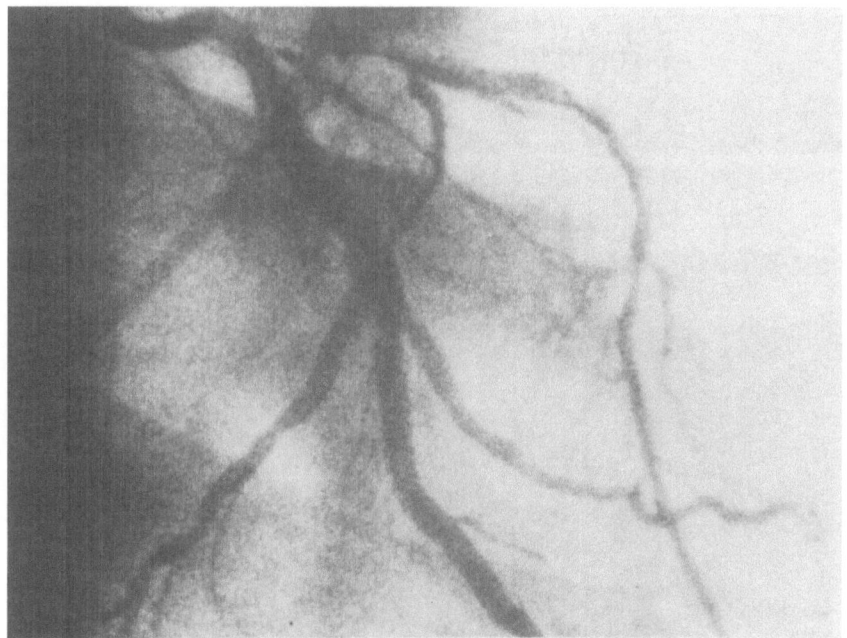

Fig. 11a.

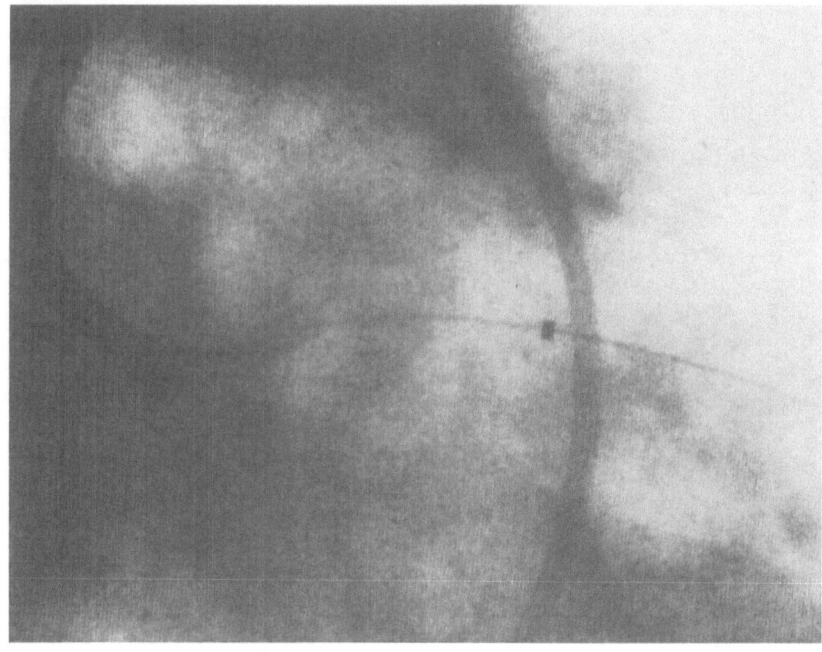

Fig. 11b.

Figs. 11 a–e. ELCA for ostial disease: a) RAO cranial projection showing total LAD lesion; b) 2.2-mm laser catheter across the lesion; c) post-ELCA; d) post adjunctive PTCA with 2.5 mm balloon; e) post-ELCA and adjunctive PTCA.

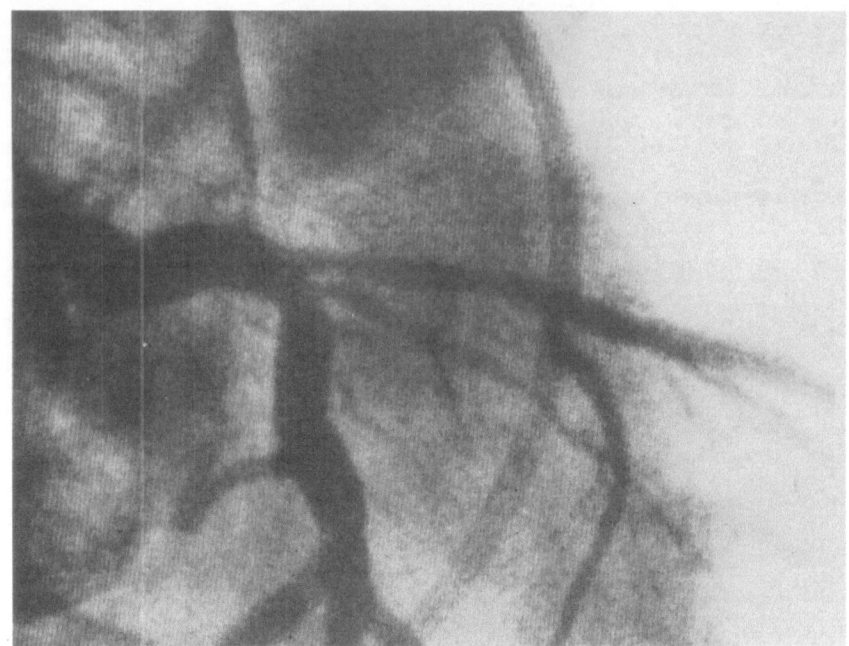

Fig. 11c.

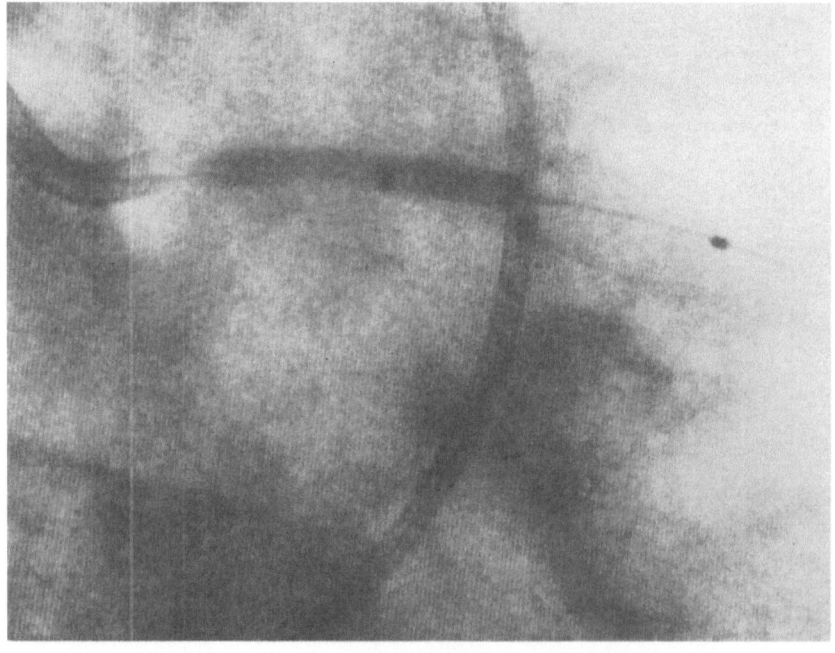

Fig. 11d.

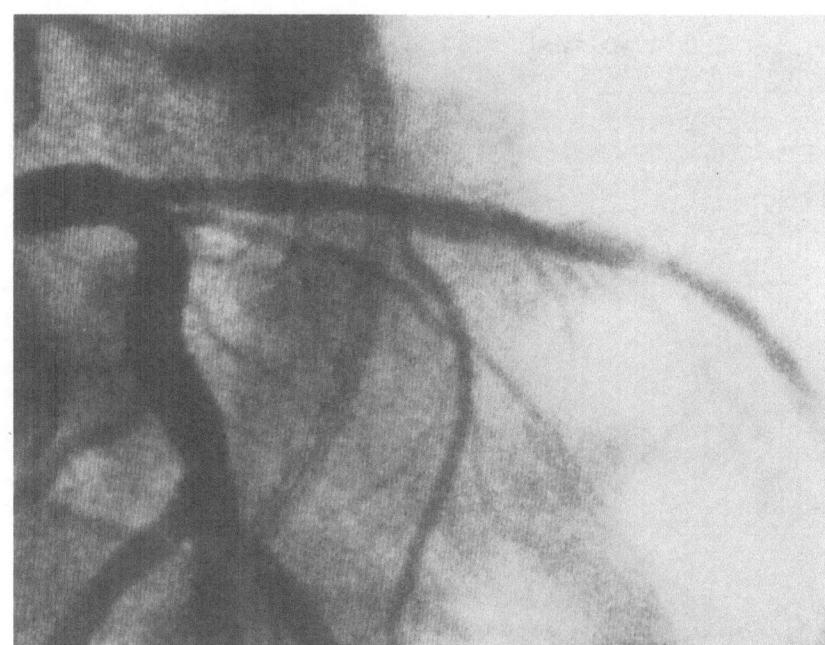

Fig. 11e.

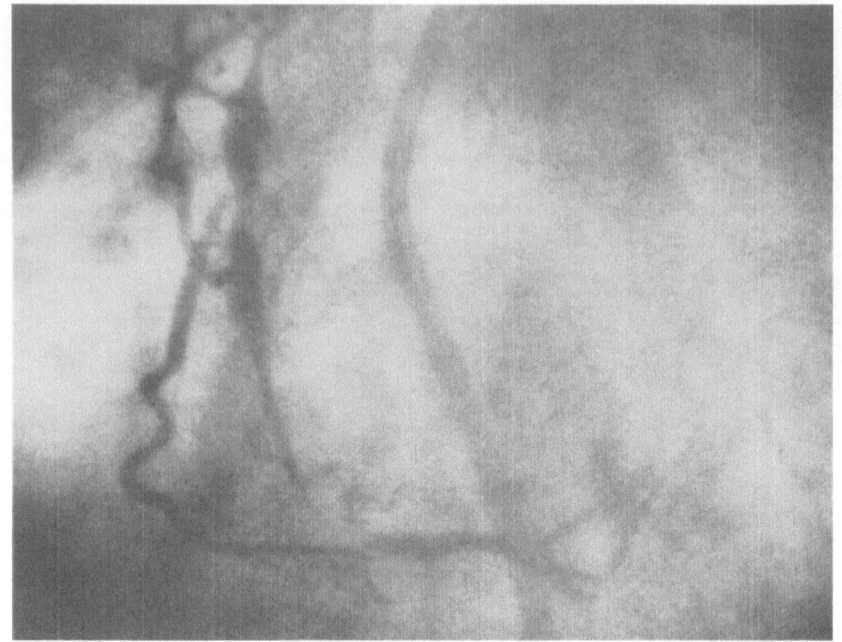

Fig. 12a.

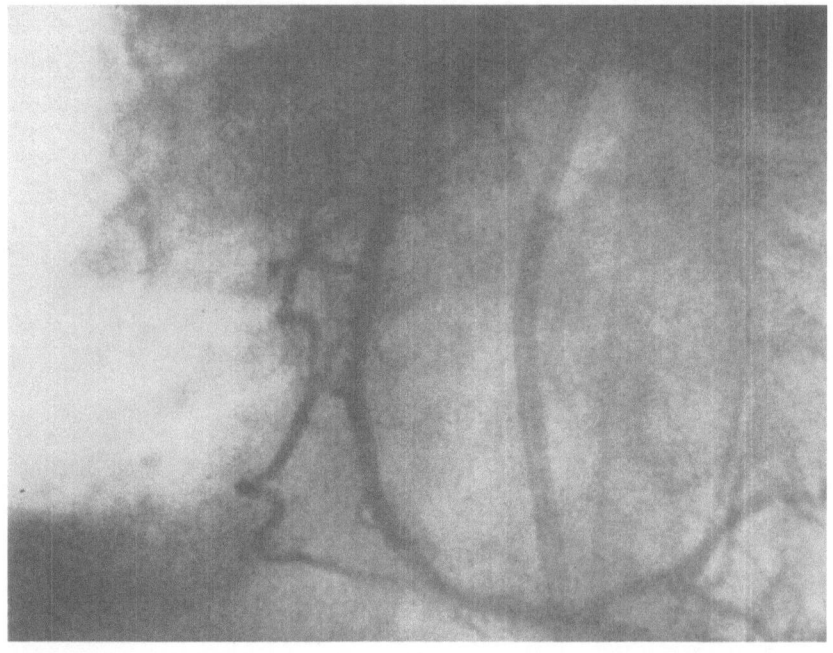

Fig. 12b.

Figs. 12 a–c. a) Totally occluded RCA in LAO projection; b) post ELCA; c) post adjunctive PTCA.

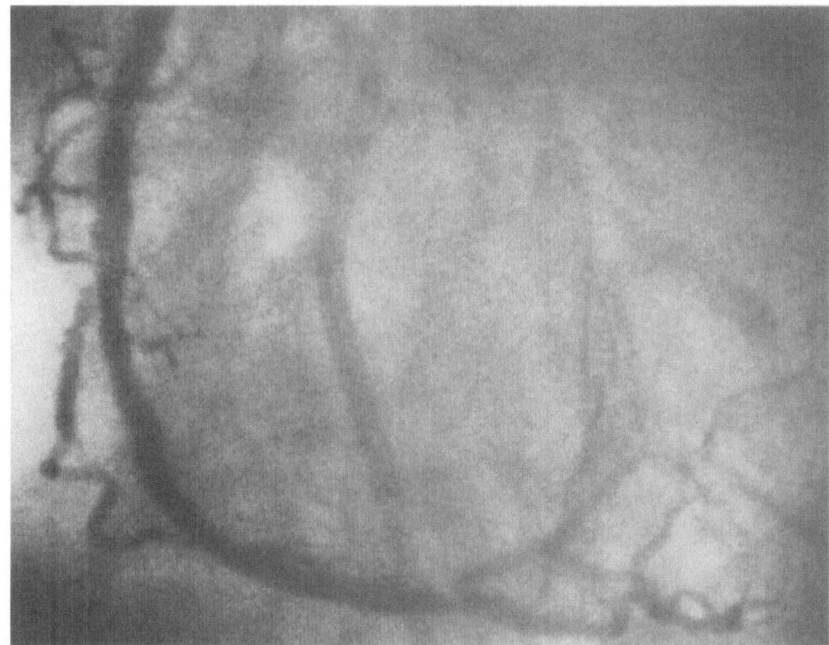

Fig. 12c.

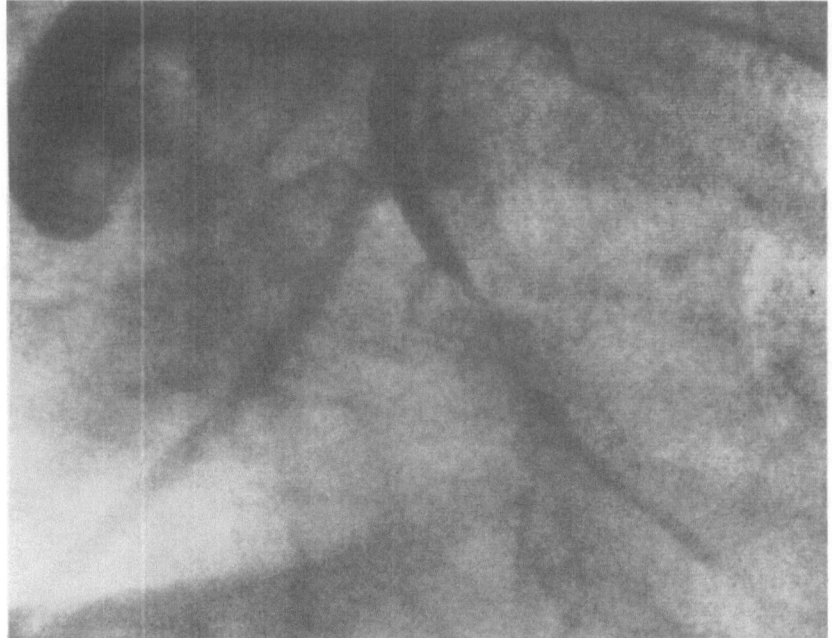

Fig. 13a.

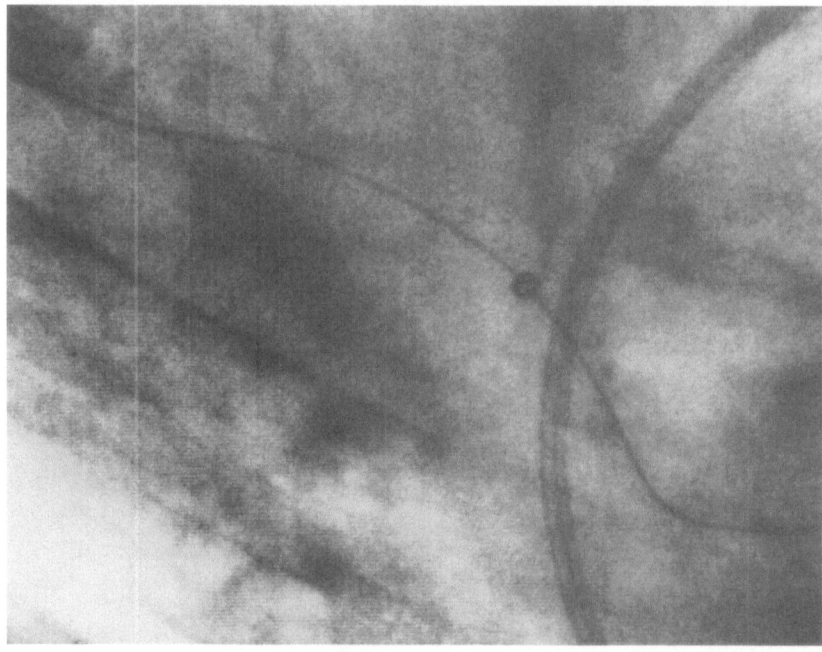

Fig. 13b.

Figs. 13 a–d. a) LAO angiogram of severe restenosis of LCX 5 months after PTCA; b) 2.0 mm laser catheter across lesion; c) immediately post-stand-alone ELCA with 2.0 mm catheter; d) 6-months post-ELCA.

96

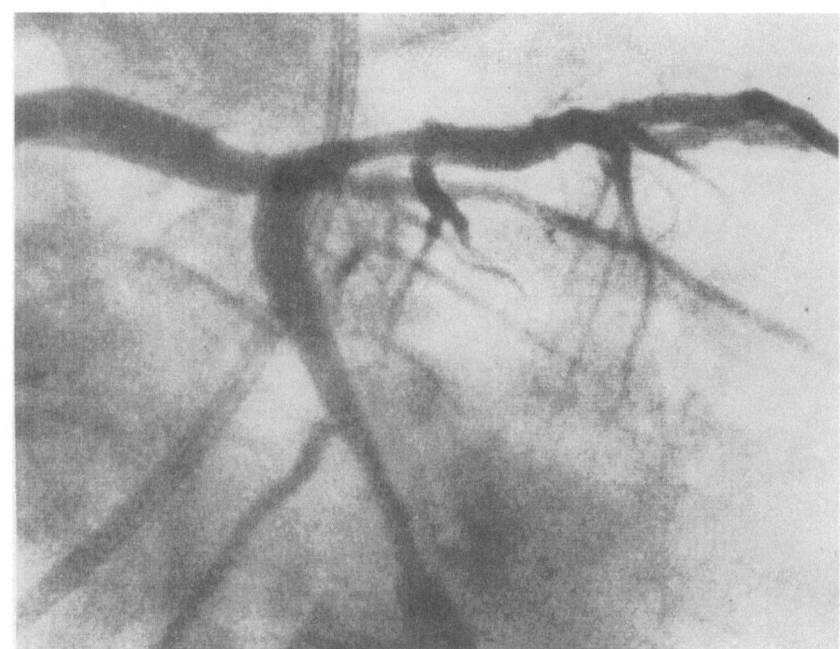

Fig. 13c.

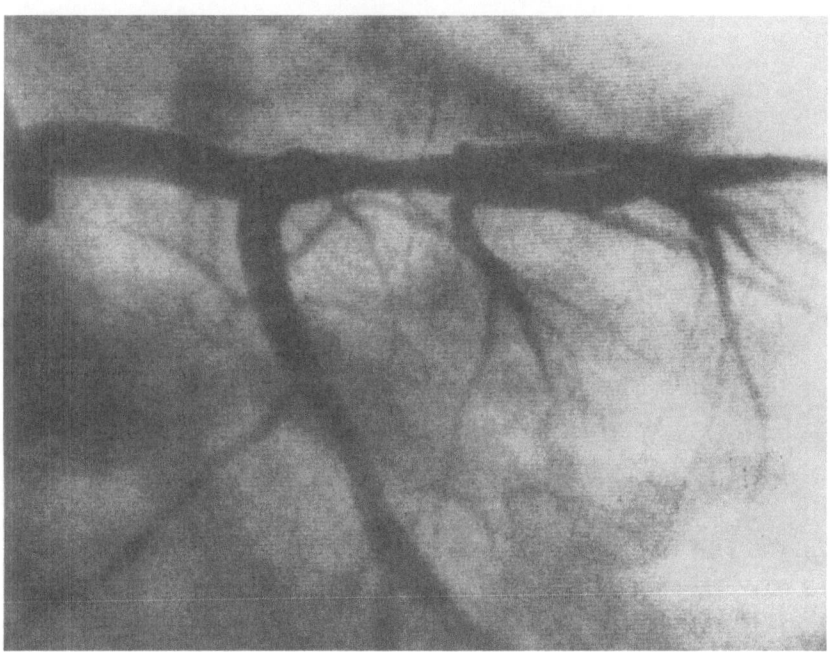

Fig. 13d.

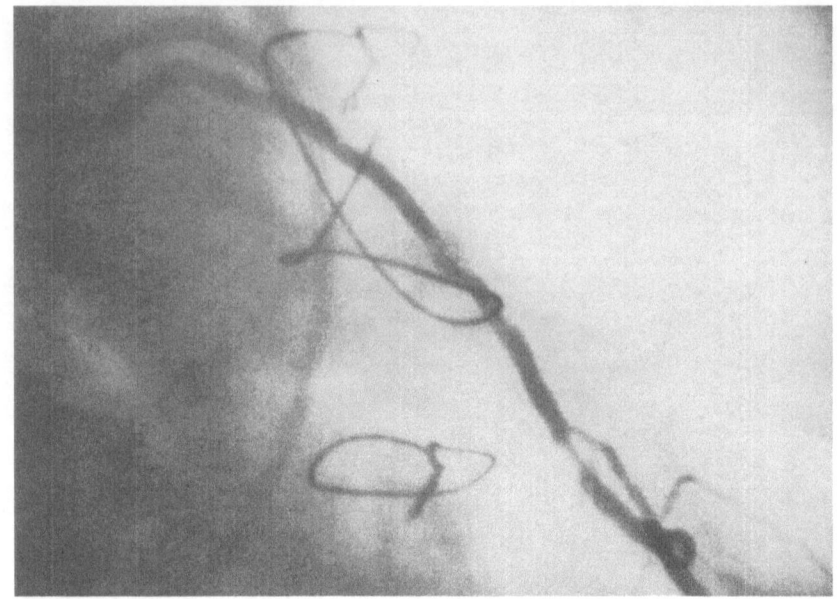

Fig. 14a.

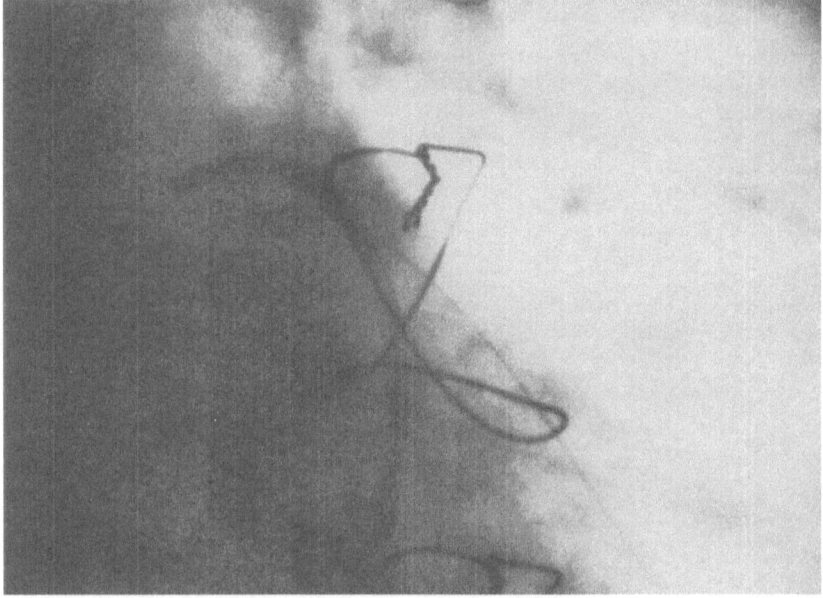

Fig. 14b.

Figs. 14a–c. a) RAO angiogram of severe lesion in SVG to LAD; b) 2.0-mm laser catheter across the lesion; c) post-stand alone ELCA.

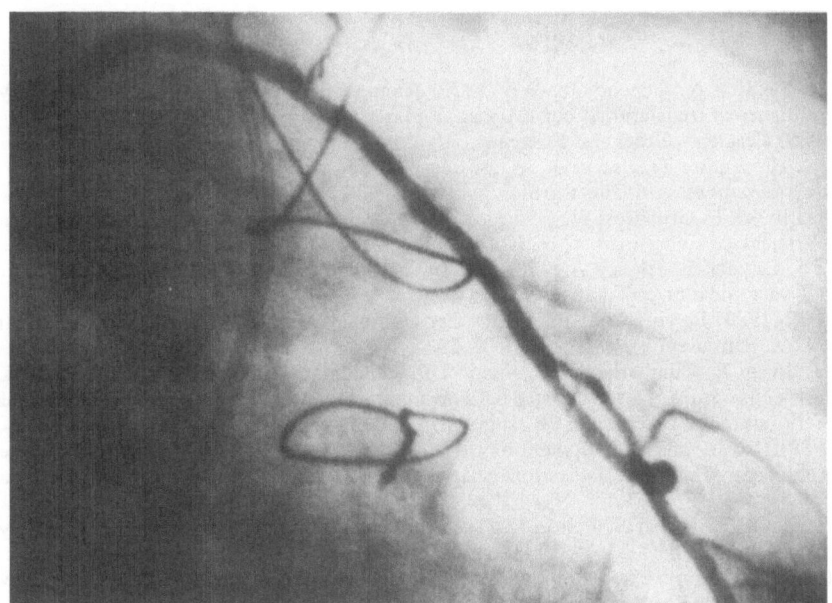

Fig. 14c.

References

1. Gruntzig AR, Senning A, Siegenthaler WE (1979) Nonoperative dilatation of coronary artery stenosis: Percutaneous transluminal coronary angioplasty. New Engl J Med 301: 61
2. Waller B (1989) Crackers, Breakers, Stretchers, Drillers, Scrapers, Shavers, Burners, Welders and Melters – The Future Treatment of Atherosclerotic Coronary Artery Disease? A Clinical-Morphologic Assessment. Am Coll Cardiology 1: 969–987
3. Forrester JS, Litvack F, Grundfest W, Hickey A (1987) A per-spective of coronary disease seen through the arteries of living man. Circulation 75: 505–513
4. Grundfest WS, Litvack F, Hickey A et al. (1987) The current status of angioscopy and laser angioplasty. J vasc Surg 5: 667–673
5. Litvack F et al. (1989) Percutaneous Excimer Laser Coronary Angioplasty in Lesions Not Well Suited for PTCA. Circulation 80 (suppl II): II–253
6. Sanborn TA, Bonan R, Cumberland DC, Faxon DP, Leachman R, Linnemeier TJ, Myler RK (1988) Percutaneous coronary laser-assisted balloon angioplasty with flexible, central lumen laser probe catheters (abstract). Circulation 78 (suppl II): II–295
7. White G (1989) History and development of cardiovascular endoscopy. In: White GH, White RA (eds.) Angioscopy: Vascular and coronary applications. Year Book Medical Publ, Chicago pp 20–36
8. Block PC, Myler RK, Stertzer S, Fallon JT (1981) Morphology after transluminal angioplasty in human beings. New Engl J Med 305: 382–385
9. Waller BF (1987) Pathology of transluminal balloon angioplasty used in the treatment of coronary heart disease. Hum Path 18: 476–484
10. Waller, BF (1983) Early and late morphologic changes in human coronary arteries after percutaneous transluminal coronary angioplasty. Clin Cardiol 6: 363–372
11. Linnemeier RJ, Bonan R, Cumberland DC, Faxon DP, Leachman R, Myler RK, Sanborn TA (1988) Human percutaneous laser-assisted coronary angioplasty of saphenous vein bypass grafts: Early multicenter experience (abstract). Circulation 78 (suppl II): II–295
12. Crea F, Davies G, McKenna W, Pashazade M, Taylor K, Maser A (1986) Percutaneous laser recanalization of coronary arteries. Lancet 1: 214–215
13. Litvack F, Grundfest WS, Segalowitz J, Papoionanniou T, Goldenberg T, Laudenslager J, Hestrin L, Forrester JS, Eigler N, Cook S (1990) Interventional cardiovascular therapy by laser and thermal angioplasty. Circulation 81 (suppl IV): IV–109–IV–116
14. Litvack F et al. (1988) Role of Laser and Thermal Ablation Devices in the Treatment of Vascular Diseases. AM J Cardiol 61: 81G–86G
15. Eldar M (1989) Laser angioplasty: a review. Review Article: 68 REFS. Isr J Med Sci 25: 222–228
16. Schaldach M (1990) Cardiovascular laser application. Review Article: 30 REFS. Artif Orsans 14: 28–40
17. Boulnais JL (1986) Photophysical processes in recent medical laser developments: A review. Lasers Med Sci 1: 47–66
18. Cote G (1989) Catheter systems for laser angioplasty. In: Abela GS (ed.) Lasers in cardiovascular medicine and surgery: Fundamentals and techniques. Kluwer, Norwell, MA
19. Steg G, Rongione AJ, Gal D, DeJesus ST, Clarke RH, Isner JM (1988) Contrasting effects of continuous wave versus pulsed laser irradiation on vascular smooth muscle (abstract). Lasers Surg Med 8: 152
20. Avrillier S, Ollivier JP, Gandjbakhch I, Delettre E, Bussiere JL (1990) XeCl excimer laser coronary angioplasty: a convergence of favourable factors. Review Article: 24 REFS. J Photochem Photobiol B 6 (1–2): 249–257
21. Grundfest WS, Segalowitz J, Goldenberg T et al. (1990) The Effect of Fiber Optic Delivery System Geometry, Power Desity and Energy on Excimer Laser Luminal Recanalization. Circulation 82 (suppl IV): III–495
22. Abela GS, Normann S, Cohen D, Feldman RL, Geiser EA, Conti CR (1982) Effects of carbon dioxide, Nd-YAG, and argon laser radiation on coronary atheromatous plaques. Amer J Cardiol 50: 1199–1205
23. Grundfest WS, Litvack F, Forrester JS et al. (1985) "Laser Ablation of Human Atherosclerotic Plaque Without Adjacent Tissue Injury." AM J Cardiol 53: 929–933

24. Litvack F et al. (1987) Comparison of Acute and Chronic Effects of Argon and excimer Laser Energy on Canine Aorta. J Am Coll Cardiol: 178A
25. Diethrich EB, Hanafy HM, Santiago OJ, Bahadir I, Kiesslins JJ, Stern LA (1990) Intraoperative coronary excimer laser angioplasty: Preliminary Clinical Experience. Angiology 41 (9 Pt 2): 777-784
26. Litvack F, Eisler NL, Margolis JR, Grundfest WS, Rothbaum D, Linnemeier T, Hestrin LB, Tsoi D, Cook SL, Krauthamer D et al. (1990) Percutaneous excimer laser coronary angioplasty. Am J Cardiol 66 (15): 1027-1032
27. Ollivier JP, Gandjbakhch I, Avrillier S, Delettre E, Bussiere JL, Cabrol C (1990) Intraoperative coronary artery endarterectomy with excimer laser. J Thorac Cardiovasc Sur 100 (4): 606-611
28. Hickey A et al. (1989) Arterial Color Flow Duplex Sonography of the Lower Extremities Before and After Excimer Laser Angioplasty. J Am Coll Cardiol Vol 13: 149A
29. Sanborn TA, Alexopoulos D, Marmur JD, Kahn H, Badimon JJ, Badimon L, Fuster V (1990) Coronary excimer laser angioplasty: reduced complications and indium-111 platelet accumulation compared with thermal laser angioplasty. J Am Coll Cardiol 16: 502-506
30. Laudenslager J et al. (1989) Design Considerations for a Clinical XeCl Excimer Laser Angioplasty System. SPIE 1066: 252-254
31. Litvack F et al. (1988) Pulsed Laser Angioplasty: Wavelength Power and Energy Dependencies Relevant to Clinical Application. Lasers in Surgery and Medicine 8: 60-65
32. Goldenberg T et al. (1989) Percutaneous Excimer Laser Angioplasty in Humans. Proxeedings of the Society of Photo-Optical Instrumentation Engineers. SPIE 1067, January 1989
33. Grundfest WS, Litvack F, Goldenberg T et al. (1985) Pulsed Ultraviolet Lasers and the Potential for Safe Laser Angioplasty. Am J Surg 150: 220-226
34. Laudenslager J et al. (1986) Effect of 308 nm Laser Pulse Duration on Fiber-optic Transmission and Biologic Tissue Ablation. Proc CLEO Paper TUA2, San Francisco, CA
35. Bresnahan DR, Bresnahan JF et al. (1990) Excimer Laser Coronary Angioplasty: Single Center Experience in Patients with anatomy suitable for Coronary Balloon Angioplasty. Circulation 82 (suppl III): III-672
36. Ghazzal ZMB, Hearn JA, Goldenberg T et al. (1990) Outcome Predictors after Excimer Laser: Detailed Multicenter Angiographic Analysis. Circulation 82 (suppl III): III-670
37. Cook S et al. Percutaneous Excimer Laser coronary Angioplasty of Lesions Not Favorable for Balloon Angioplasty. Division of Cardiology, Dept. of Medicine, Cedars-Sinai Medical Center
38. Karsch KR, Haase KK, Mauser M, Ickrath O, Voelker W, Duda S, Seipel L (1989) Percutaneous coronary excimer laser angioplasty: initial clinical results. Lancet 16; 2 (8664): 647-650
39. Eigler N et al. (1990) Excimer Laser Angioplasty of Ostial Coronary Stenosis: Results of Multicenter Study. Circulation 82 (suppl III): III-1
40. Raizner A, Litvack F, Goldenberg T et al. (1990) Improved Results in Patients with Long Coronary Stenoses Using Excimer Laser Angioplasty. Circulation 82 (suppl III): III-671
41. Reeer GS, Bresnahan JF, Bresnahan DR (1990) Excimer Laser Coronary Angioplasty (ELCA) in Patients with Restenosis after Prior Balloon Angioplasty (BA). Circulation 82 ((suppl III): III-672
42. Levine S, Mehta S, Krauthamer D, Margolis RJ (1991) Excimer Laser Coronary Angioplasty of Clacified Lesions. Abstract Am Coll Cardiology, 40th Annual Scientific Session, 1991
43. Litvack F, Grundfest WS, Goldenberg T, Laudenslager J, Forrester JS (1989) Percutaneous excimer laser angioplasty of aortocoronary saphenous vein grafts. J Am Coll Cardiol 14 (3): 803-808
44. Litvack F, Grundfest W, Eisler N, Tsoi D, Goldenberg T, Laudenslager J, Forrester J (1989) Percutaneous excimer laser coronary angioplasty (letter). Lancet 8; 2 (8654): 102
45. Untereker W, Litvack F, Margolis J et al. (1990) Excimer Laser Coronary Angioplasty of Saphenous Vein Grafts. Circulation 82 (suppl III): III-680
46. Cook S, Eigler N et al. (1990) Angiographic Determinants of Successful Excimer Laser Coronary angioplasty. Circulation 82 (suppl III): III-671
47. Karsch KR, Haase KK, Voelker W, Baumbach A, Mauser M, Seipel L (1990) Percutaneous coronary excimer laser angioplasty in patients with stable and unstable angina pectoris. Acute results and incidence of restenosis during 6-month follow-up. Comments in: Circulation: 2018-2021; Circulation 81: 1849-1859

48. Karsch KR, Haase KK, Mauser M, Voelker W (1989) Initial angiographic results in ablation of atherosclerotic plaque by percutaneous coronary excimer laser angioplasty without subsequent balloon dilation. Am J Cardiol 64 (19): 1253–1257
49. Kaltenbach M, Vallbracht C, Kober G (1987) Long Wire Technique: experience with 100 procedures. Z Kardiol 76 (suppl 6): 53–57
50. Gregory KW, Walsh AA, Schomacker KT, Kochevar IE (1990) Excimer Laer Energy Absorbed by Radiographic Contrast Media Results in Cytotoxic Photoproducts. Circulation 82 (suppl III)
51. Grundfest W. Personal Communication
52. Margolis JR, Litvack F, Krauthamer D, Trautwein R, Goldenberg T, Grundfest W (1990) Excimer laser coronary angioplasty: American multicenter experience. Herz 15: 223–232
53. Trautwein R, Margolis J et al. (1990) Excimer Laser Coronary Angioplasty of Chronic Total Occlusions. Circulation 82 (suppl III): III–687
54. Litvack F et al. (1989) Complications During Excimer Laser Angioplasty are Similar to Those During PTCA. Circulation 80 (suppl II): II–254

Authors' address:
James R. Margolis, M. D.
South Miami Hospital
Cardiovascular Laboratory
7400 S. W., 62nd Avenue
Miami, Florida 33143
USA

Coronary Excimer Laser Angioplasty: The Spectranetics Registry

T. A. Sanborn, J. A. Bittl, R. A. Hershman, R. M. Siegel

Division of Cardiology, Department of Medicine, Mount Sinai Medical Center, New York, NY in association with The New York Cardiac Center, Englewood Cliffs, New Jersey, USA

After a decade of experimental and clinical investigation, it appears that there is finally some evidence suggesting that lasers may have a role in the treatment of some patients with obstructive coronary artery disease. While not yet published, as of this writing, preliminary results from two separate registries indicate that at least one laser, the excimer laser, used either alone or in combination with conventional balloon angioplasty may have a benefit in the treatment of long lesions, greater than 20 mm, by increasing the success rate and decreasing the complication rate in these complex lesions. The present review will summarize the initial clinical experience with the Spectranetics Excimer Laser Angioplasty System.

Initial Clinical Experience

Rationale

As an over-the-wire device, the excimer laser catheters are currently only being used on coronary artery stenoses or occlusions that can be crossed with a guidewire. Like atherectomy, excimer laser angioplasty is testing the hypothesis that removal of atheroma − in this case by laser ablation − will result in less restenosis than occurs with balloon angioplasty. By leaving behind a smoother luminal surface without the deep arterial injury or a "scalloping" effect of atherectomy, excimer laser angioplasty may lead to less restenosis. To date, however, only a few case reports and small clinical series have been published on percutaneous coronary excimer laser angioplasty with very little follow-up data [1–8]. Furthermore, as is evident from these reports, a wide range of catheter sizes and different laser parameters are under investigation in these early feasibility trials. Thus, long-term follow-up with a high percentage of angiography analysis will be required to address the question of whether excimer laser angioplasty has any effect on restenosis.

Excimer laser angioplasty may also have a role in treating lesions that may be difficult or impossible to treat with conventional balloon angioplasty. This hypothesis also awaits additional studies.

Pre-treatment

Patients selected for percutaneous coronary excimer laser angioplasty are treated essentially the same as those undergoing conventional balloon angioplasty in terms of their medications (aspirin, calcium channel blockers, 10000–15000 heparin bolus, intracoronary nigtroglycerin), guiding catheters, and guidewires.

Guidewire selection

As in conventional balloon angioplasty, guidewires with a distal radioopaque tip and a more proximal radiolucent section are preferred for excimer laser angioplasty as the lesion can be better visualized before, during, and after laser treatment. Both 0.014- and 0.018-inch guidewires have been used with some benefit in providing more support, and "straightening" of the coronary artery seen with the 0.018-inch guidewire. A customized "laserwire" (Advanced Catheter Systems) also exist which is 0.018-inches in diameter and is firmer up to the last few centimeters of a floppy distal tip. Whether this additional thickness is necessary to help keep the laser catheter coaxial in the artery remains to be determined. Other guidewires can certainly be used; however, the presence of a radiolucent section of a guidewire in the lesion being treated is most helpful in visualizing a laser effect and in observing any subtle linear dissection which would be considered a contraindication to further use of the laser.

Guiding catheter selection

For excimer laser catheters up to 1.8 mm outer diameter, conventional 8F guiding catheters can be used. Larger 2.0 mm catheters require 9F guiding catheters. In order to accommodate the greatest number of fiberoptic bundles, these laser catheters have a greater outer diameter than conventional balloon catheters. These larger laser catheter shaft sizes do not allow for much additional space inside the guiding catheter. Thus, it is more important to prevent acute angles in the guiding catheter which could cause resistance to advancement of these larger diameter laser catheters through the guiding catheter and the coronary arteries. An angiographer has to be much more careful with his guiding catheter selection and may actually have to size up from a left 4 catheter to a left 4.5 guiding catheter in order to obtain the most coaxial alignment with the left main coronary artery. The short tip (SL) guiding catheters also have some advantage as they decrease the acute angle at the end of the conventional JL guiding catheters.

Excimer laser procedure

First, a 0.014–0.018-inch guidewire is advanced across the lesion into the distal coronary artery, with its position confirmed fluoroscopically as in conventional balloon angioplasty. After extending the guidewire, the laser catheter is then advanced over the guidewire up to the lesion. Small contrast injections (3cc) confirm the position of the laser catheter in direct contact with the origin of the lesion. Next, a short 3–5 s period of laser energy delivery is used with the catheter in a stationary position and the energy fluence set at 50 mJ/mm^2. The rationale behind this initial stationary attempt is to initiate lesion ablation before advancement of the catheter. While unconfirmed, it is thought that this may decrease the risk of mechanical dissection of the artery. After this initial stationary step, the excimer laser catheter is then slowly advanced through the lesion at a rate of 0.5–1.0 mm per second and short 3–5 s periods of laser energy delivery. Several of these laser attempts may be necessary to completely transverse the lesion. If a lesion cannot be transversed at a fluence of 50 mJ/mm^2, then the energy fluence is increased to 60 mJ/mm^2 in order to maximize laser ablation. Once a lesion has been crossed, the catheter is withdrawn (without laser delivery) back into the guiding catheter, and angiography is performed to document the results and to be sure that spasm, dissection, or perforation have not occurred. It is still unclear whether additional passes through the lesion are beneficial in providing more laser ablation or are harmful by increasing the risk of complications such as dissection or perforation. Certainly, once a catheter passes smoothly through a lesion no further laser attempts are made. After the final pass, the catheter is withdrawn completely from the guiding catheter and repeat coronary arteriography is performed to document the laser result. By protocol design, the majority of lesions are then dilated with subsequent balloon angioplasty in order to maximally reduce the luminal stenosis and to provide the greatest luminal diameter. This approach is somewhat different from other excimer laser protocols which have considered a residual lesion of less than 50% to be adequate, such that no further balloon angioplasty was performed. This latter approach may lead to a higher incidence of angiographic restenosis.

In the majority of cases, systemic heparinization is maintained overnight and sheaths are removed the following morning. Discharged medications include aspirin (325 mg/day) and other cardiac medications as prescribed by the referring physician. Systemic anticoagulation with coumadin has not been a part of this protocol.

Procedural definitions

Successful excimer laser angioplasty or laser recanalization is defined as passage of the laser catheter through the stenosis and a greater than 20% improvement of the luminal diameter stenosis (visual estimate) without perforation. Procedural success is defined as less that 50% residual stenosis without major complications of myocardial infarction (CPK > 200 mg/dl), emergency bypass surgery, or death.

Initial multicenter results

The initial clinical experience of percutaneous coronary excimer laser-assisted balloon angioplasty with the Spectranetics excimer laser catheter was recently published [8] and is briefly summarized as follows.

Acute angiographic results

The clinical and angiographic variables for this series are summarized in Table 1. Based on an intention-to-treat analysis, the excimer laser catheter was able to traverse the lesion and reduce the percent diameter stenosis by at least 20% in 138 of 158 (87%) coronary artery stenoses. Laser failure was attributed to the following: inability to cross the lesion [n = 15, due to vessel tortuosity (n = 5), low-energy fluence (n = 4), calcified lesion (n = 3), and large device profile or catheter dead space between the fibers (n = 3)]; vessel perforation (n = 3); laser generator failure (n = 1); or radiographic failure (n = 1).

In this early feasibility study with small 1.5- and 1.75-mm diameter catheters, excimer laser angioplasty was able to reduce the residual stenosis to less than 50% in

Table 1. Clinical and angiographic variables.

Clinical variables: (141 patients)

Age (years)

	Mean	60
	Range	32–84

Sex

	Male	98 (69%)
	Female	43 (31%)

Angina

	Stable	78 (55%)
	Unstable	63 (45%)

Functional class (CCS)

	I	4 (3%)
	II	16 (11%)
	III	47 (33%)
	IV	74 (53%)

Angiographic variables: (158 stenoses)

Vessel treated

	LAD	95 (60%)
	RCA	29 (18%)
	LCX	26 (16%)
	SVG	8 (5%)

Repeat angioplasty	30 (19%)
Multivessel angioplasty	15 (11%)
Severity of stenosis prior to treatment (mean + standard error)	87 + 09

CCS = Canadian Cardiovascular Society

77 of 158 (49%) lesions; however, due to protocol design to obtain the largest lumen and the greatest reduction in the stenosis only 9 of 158 (5.7%) lesions were treated with excimer angioplasty alone. An angiographic example of a patient treated with "stand-alone" excimer laser angioplasty that resulted in a smoother lumen with less dissection than on a prior attempt with balloon angioplasty is shown in Fig. 1 along with a 9-month follow-up angiogram which demonstrates no restenosis. Overall, laser-assisted balloon angioplasty was successful (residual stenosis less than 50% without major complication) in 129 of 141 (91%) patients.

Complications

Laser perforation is the most feared complication of coronary laser angioplasty, however, with the over-the-wire approach, this occured is only 3 (1.9%) attempts. Two of these cases required emergency bypass surgery while one was successfully treated with prolonged balloon inflation [9]. One diseased small diagonal side branch became

106

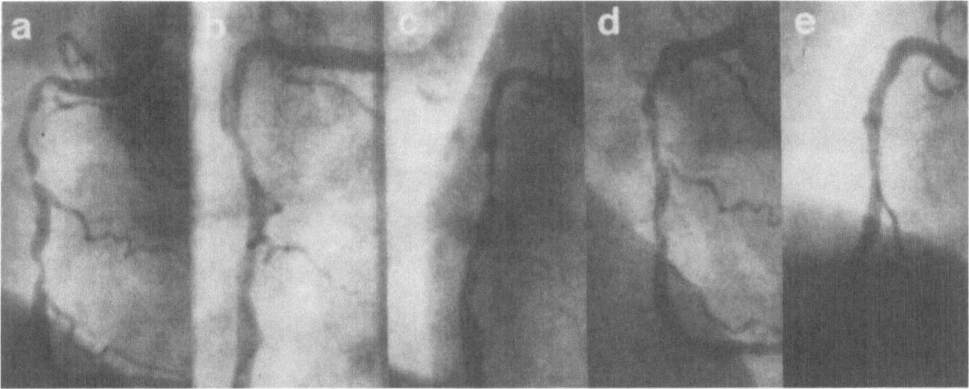

Fig. 1. Serial angiograms of a diffusely diseased right coronary artery treated with conventional balloon angioplasty and then excimer laser angioplasty alone when restenosis developed. a) Sequential 90% and 70% stenoses in a diffusely diseased vessel. b) Angiography after dilation with a 3.0 mm balloon catheter. An intimal flap persisted despite prolonged balloon inflations. c) 80% restenosis 3 months after balloon angioplasty. d) Angiogram after excimer laser angioplasty with a 1.7 mm excimer laser catheter which did not reveal any angiographic evidence of dissection. e) Follow-up angiography 9 months after excimer laser angioplasty with 15% residual stenosis. (Reproduced with permission of T. A. Sanborn and The American College of Cardiology from [8]).

occluded after five passes of the excimer laser catheter and could not be recanalized with a guidewire; this resulted in a small non-Q-wave myocardial infarction (peak CPK 381 mg/dl). These four immediate laser-related complications occurred during a modification of the catheter tip design. This design was abandoned after these four cases and no further laser perforations occurred in subsequent cases. Single episodes of vessel spasm or intraluminal filling defects seen after excimer laser angioplasty were not angina producing and were successfully treated with intracoronary nitroglycerin and balloon dilation. A summary of these complications is presented in Table 2.

While it is difficult to separate and attribute complications to either the laser or balloon angioplasty procedure when the catheters were used sequentially, those observed after balloon dilation were also low (Table 2). Except for the above-mentioned complications seen after laser attempts, the use of the laser catheter did not lead to a greater risk of performing balloon angioplasty. Three emergent or urgent bypass procedures were performed for spiral dissection (n=2) or abrupt closure (n=1) after balloon dilation. Non-Q-wave myocardial infarction was attributed to side branch occlusion (n=2), distal embolization (n=1), dissection (n=1), and abrupt closure (n=2) after balloon angioplasty. Whether excimer laser angioplasty predisposes a particular lesion to a complication after balloon dilation could not be excluded. Overall, major complications (MI, CABG, death) were observed in only 10 (7.1 %) patients as two patients had small non-Q-wave myocardial infarction despite emergency CABG.

Despite the prototype nature of these laser catheters and the fact that each investigator had to go through a learning curve with the laser angioplasty technique, complications were in the range of what has been published in recent but historic reports [10] for conventional balloon angioplasty (Table 3).

107

Table 2. Procedural complications.

	Laser-related n (%)	PTCA-related n (%)	Total n (%)
By lesion (n=158)			
Abrupt closure (<24 h)	0	2 (1.3)	2 (1.3)
Branch occlusion	1 (0.6)	2 (1.3)	3 (1.9)
Dissection	0	10 (6.3)	10 (6.3)
Embolization	0	2 (1.3)	2 (1.3)
Filling defect	1 (0.6)	1 (0.6)	2 (1.3)
Perforation	3 (1.9)	0	3 (1.9)
Spasm	1 (0.6)	1 (0.6)	2 (1.3)
By patient (n=141)			
MI (CPK>200)	1 (0.7)	6 (4.3)	7 (4.8)
Emergency CABG	2 (1.4)	3 (2.1)	5 (3.5)
Death	0	0	0
			10 (7.1)

Table 3. Procedural complications.

	NHLBI PTCA Registry* (1801 patients)	Coronary excimer laser-assisted angioplasty (141 patients)
Abrupt closure	4.9%	1.4%
Branch occlusion	2.1%	2.1%
Dissection	4.8%	7.1%
Spasm	1.3%	1.4%
MI	4.3%	5.0%
Emergency CABG	3.5%	3.5%
Death	1.0%	0%

*Holmes et al. (1988) J Am Coll Cardiol 12: 1149–1155

Clinical follow-up

In early clinical follow-up of 1 to 10 months (mean of 7 months), patients treated with coronary excimer laser angioplasty did not demonstrate any increase in clinical recurrence of symptoms: however, the follow-up has been short. To date, 111 of 141 (79%) patients remain asymptomatic while symptoms of angina have recurred in a total of 27 of 141 (19%) patients. Of the small number of patients who have reached 6-month follow-up, restenosis has occurred in 7 of 24 (29%) patients; however, these patients were treated early in this series when laser parameters, delivery catheters, and operator technique were being developed. There have been three deaths in this series; one after emergency bypass surgery, one after elective bypass surgery for dissection after balloon angioplasty, and one after elective PTCA of another vessel.

Evolving excimer laser equipment and technique

During this initial trial there was considerable evolution and modification of the laser catheters as well as the actual laser angioplasty technique. For example, it was determined that greater recanalization success occurred at an energy fluence of 50–60 mJ/mm^2 as opposed to the initial 30 mJ/mm^2 [7–8]. In addition, some of the laser failures were due to the prototype nature of the laser delivery system which improved in flexibility by using 100 μm as opposed to 200 μm fiberoptics. However, many other questions remain to be answered which are related to catheter development (tip size and shape, optimal number of fibers with least amount of catheter dead space, flexibility, trackability, guidewire selection), the ideal laser parameters (fluence, repetition rate, pulse duration) and operator techniques (number of passes, rate of advancement through the lesion, etc). These questions are just now being addressed. Currently, larger 2.0 mm laser catheters are being evaluated that are capable of producing larger channels to obviate the requirement for follow-up balloon angioplasty [11]. These improved catheters will allow for more independent analysis of excimer laser angioplasty alone. Whether there will be a benefit of "debulking" a lesion with excimer laser-assisted balloon angioplasty will require a randomized trial comparing acute and follow-up results to balloon angioplasty alone. Preliminary quantitative angiographic analysis suggests that if the laser is able to reduce the lesion to less than 30% residual stenosis, then the incidence of restenosis was reduced [12].

Better angioplasty?

Figure 1 is a representative angiographic example of an observation made numerous times in this study, i. e., the angiographic result after excimer laser angioplasty appeared to result in less vessel dissection than that often seen after conventional balloon angioplasty. While it is difficult to prove that excimer laser angioplasty resulted in a smoother lumen than balloon dilation using angiography alone, it will be interesting to analyze the incidence of complications as more cases are performed by excimer laser angioplasty alone without subsequent balloon angioplasty. Intraluminal ultrasound may be able to determine whether this impression of a "smoother" channel does exist after excimer laser recanalization as compared to the fracture and dissection of balloon dilation.

Future directions

The feasibility of excimer laser angioplasty and excimer laser-assisted balloon angioplasty has been demonstrated in several clinical registries. There is some preliminary data that this technique may have its initial application in improving the success rate and reducing complications for angioplasty of long diffuse stenoses greater than 20 mm. There are still many questions regarding the optimal operator techniques as well as the actual laser catheters which will require significant evaluation and modifications in the near future. Catheter-related issues will center on such aspects as flexibility, trackability, profile, and maximal ablative potential. There is also a need to create larger laser channels safely. Whether the latter will require larger sized catheters or can be accomplished by positioning the catheter to one side of the vessel

109

or another as in directional atherectomy remains to be determined. Hopefully, with greater clinical experience, there will be answers to these questions.

References

1. Litvack F, Grundfest W, Eigler N, Tsoi B, Goldenberg T, Laudenslager J, Forrester J (1989) Percutaneous excimer laser coronary angioplasty. Lancet II: 102–103
2. Sanborn TA, Hershman RA, Torre SR, Sherman W, Cohen M, Ambrose JA (1989) Percutaneous excimer laser coronary angioplasty. Lancet II: 616
3. Karsch KR, Haase KK, Mauser M, Ickrath O, Voelker W, Duda S, Seipel L (1989) Percutaneous coronary excimer laser angioplasty: Initial clinical results. Lancet II: 647–650
4. Litvack F, Grundfest WS, Goldenberg T, Laudenslager J, Forrester JS (1989) Percutaneous excimer laser angioplasty of aortocoronary saphenous vein grafts. J Am Coll Cardiol 14: 803–808
5. Karsch KR, Haase KK, Mauser M, Voelker W (1989) Initial angiographic results in ablation of atherosclerotic plaque by percutaneous coronary excimer laser angioplasty without subsequent balloon dilatation. Am J Cardiol 64: 1253–1257
6. Karsch KR, Haase KK, Voelker W, Baumbach A, Mauser M, Seipel L (1990) Percutaneous coronary excimer laser angioplasty in patients with stable and unstable angina pectoris: acute results and incidence of restenosis during 6-month follow-up. Circulation 81: 1849–1859
7. Sanborn TA, Torre SR, Sharma SK, Hershman RA, Cohen M, Sherman W, Ambrose JA (1991) Percutaneous coronary excimer laser-assisted angioplasty: initial clinical and quantitative angiographic results in 50 patients. J Am Coll Cardiol 17: 94–99
8. Sanborn TA, Bittl JA, Hershman RA, Siegel RM (1991) Percutaneous coronary excimer laser-assited angioplasty: initial multicenter experience in 141 patients. J Am Coll Cardiol 17: 169B–173B
9. Parker JD, Ganz P, Selwyn AP, Bittl JA (1991) Successful treatment of an excimer laser-associated coronary artery perforation with the Stack perfusion catheter. Cath Cardiovasc Diagn 22: 118–123
10. Holmes DR. Jr., Holubkov MS, Vlietstra RE, Kelsey SF, Reeder GS, Dorros G, William DO, Cowley MJ, Faxon DP, KLent KM, Bentivoglio LG, Detre K, and the co-investigators of the National Heart, Lung, and Blood Institute (1988) Percutaneous Transluminal Coronary Angioplasty Registry. Comparison of complications during percutaneous transluminal coronary angioplasty from 1977 to 1981 and from 1985 to 1986: The National Heart, Lung and Blood Institute Percutaneous Transluminal Coronary Angioplasty Registry. J AmColl Cardiol 12: 1149–1155
11. Torre SR, Sanborn TA, Sharma SK, Cohen M, Ambrose JA (1990) Percutaneous coronary excimer laser angioplasty: quantitative angiographic analysis demonstrates improved angioplasty results with larger laser catheters. Circulation 82: III–671
12. Sanborn TA, Bittl JA, Torre SR (1991) Procedural success, in-hospital events, and follow-up clinical and angiographic results of percutaneous coronary excimer laser-assisted angioplasty. J Am Coll Cardiol 17: 206A

Authors' address:
Timothy A. Sanborn, M. D.
Division of Cardiology
Box 1030
Mount Sinai Medical Center
One Gustave L. Levy Place
New York, NY 10029, USA

The European Experience
Coronary Excimer Laser Angioplasty: The Technolas Study Group

K. K. Haase, A. Baumbach, K. R. Karsch

Med. Klinik III, Tübingen, FRG

Introduction

Coronary artery disease accounts for approximately 80–90% of heart disease, which is today the leading cause of morbidity and mortality in industrialized nations. The number of deaths from heart disease has been reported to be declining from the 1970s, a fact that is largely attributable to a decrease in mortality from coronary artery disease [3]. New possibilities of acute and long-term management of patients with coronary artery disease have contributed to this decrease in mortality.

Medical, interventional, and surgical techniques are the three therapeutic options for patients with disabling symptoms of angina pectoris. The two current gold standards for revascularization are coronary artery bypass grafting (CABG) and percutaneous transluminal coronary angioplasty (PTCA). If experimental atherosclerosis is subjected to balloon angioplasty, it may result in organized thrombus formation and smooth muscle cell proliferation with a maximum of mitotic activity as early as 7 days after intervention [6]. Balloon dilatation results in initial arterial overdistension, splitting of the neointimal cap of the atheroma, stretching of the vessel, and compression of the atheroma [1]. It is suspected that the extent of injury of vessel wall tissue correlates with the incidence of restenosis, which is approximately 20–40% [4, 12, 15]. This unacceptable high rate of restenotic lesions is the major cause for the search for new techniques to reduce atherosclerotic plaque.

Since excimer laser angioplasty is thought to remove the atherosclerotic lesion rather than remodeling it, it was expected that the extent of vessel wall injury may be reduced. In March 1989, a study was initiated in a first series of patients using a 1.4-mm diameter prototype laser catheter device to ablate obstructive lesions in native coronary arteries [10, 11]. In a second and third series of patients the transmission device was improved in regard to flexibility, diameter variability, and trackability. Additionally, the pulse duration of the excimer laser was increased from 60 ns to 115 ns in the third series of patients, resulting in an improved energy transmission via the optical wave-guides.

In this chapter, we report on the acute clinical results and the 6-month follow-up in all three series of patients.

Methods

Laser and transmission devices

A commercial xenon chloride excimer laser (Technolas Inc., MAX-10, Munich, FRG) emitting energy at a wavelength of 308 nm with a pulse duration of 60 ns was used.

The laser was operated at a repetition rate of 20 Hertz. The laser energy was coupled into unshielded quartz fibers with core diameters of 100 μm each. For the first series of patients a prototype 1.4 mm laser catheter with a concentric arrangement of 20 quartz fibers was used. Through a central lumen (of the device) a 0.014-inch guide wire could easily be moved backward and forward, enabling an over-the-wire laser process. Fixation of the catheter system was performed at the proximal and distal ends only to guarantee maximal catheter shaft flexibility. A gold marker at the fiber tip allowed visualization during angiography and intervention.

In the second and third series of patients, improved laser catheters were available. Improvement was achieved in flexibility, diameter variability, and trackability. A 1.3 mm laser catheter contained 20 quartz fibers, a 1.5 mm catheter 30 fibers, and a 1.8 mm laser catheter 36 fibers. In comparison to the catheter devices of the first series the length of the stiff and inflexible tip was decreased from 6–9 mm to 2–3 mm. Additionally, a longer pulse duration, increased from 60 to 115 ns, was used in the third series of patients, resulting in a better energy transmission down the quartz fibers. Energy transmission was measured with a commercial power meter prior to laser irradiation and after lesion treatment. The energy density measured at the catheter tip was 30 ± 5 mJ/mm2 in the first series, 42 ± 14 mJ/mm2 in the second series, and 67 ± 19 mJ/mm2 in the third series. Total irradiation time was 123 ± 65 s, 117 ± 72 s, and 51 ± 27 s for series 1, 2, and 3, respectively. The patency of the fibers for light transmission was determined by visual inspection of the catheter tip before and after intervention.

Patient populations

A total of 147 patients was enrolled in the study of coronary excimer laser angioplasty, from March 1989, to October 1990.

All patients had been previously selected for PTCA on the basis of symptoms and angiographic findings. Forty-nine of the 60 patients of the first series were markedly limited by severe exertional angina pectoris, despite medical therapy, and 11 patients had unstable angina with reversible ST-segment changes at rest, despite therapy with nitroglycerin, β-blocking agents, and calcium antagonists. Patients with angiographic evidence of intracoronary thrombi or evolving myocardial infarction were excluded.

Due to the unfavorable results of coronary laser angioplasty in patients with unstable angina pectoris, unstable patients were excluded in the second series of 40 patients and in the third series of 47 patients. The left anterior descending artery was the target vessel in 43/28/31 patients, the circumflex artery in 7/3/3 patients, and the right coronary artery in 10/9/14 patients of series 1, 2, and 3, respectively. The baseline characteristics of all patients of series 1, 2, and 3 are depicted in Tables 1, 2, and 3.

The protocol of excimer laser angioplasty was approved by the Institutional Review Board Committee at the University of Tübingen, and informed consent was obtained from each patient before intervention.

Study protocol

The patients were prepared for excimer laser angioplasty with standard angioplasty techniques via the transfemoral approach. All patients were maintained on long-term acetylsalicylic acid (100–500 mg/daily). After a heparin bolus (10 000 units given intra-

Table 1. Patient population (first series).

		(n)
Total		60
Gender	M	49
	F	11
Mean age (years)		59 ± 11
Extent CAD	1-VD	41
	2-VD	13
	3-VD	6
Target vessel	LAD	43
	CIRC	7
	RCA	10
Lesion morphology		
-eccentric		38
-concentric		8
-occlusion		10
-long segmental		4
Lesion length		
> 10 mm		16
< 10 mm		44
CCS	1	2
	2	26
	3	21
	4	11

M = male;   F = female;   CAD = coronary   artery   disease;
VD = vessel   disease;   LAD = left   anterior   descending;
Circ = circumflex   artery;   RCA = right   coronary   artery;
CCS = Canadian Cardiovascular Society

arterially), the lesion site was visualized, and intracoronary nitroglycerin (100 µg) was administered. With a 9-French large-lumen guiding catheter placed in the ostium of the target vessel, the 0.014 inch-diameter flexible guide wire was advanced across the lesion and its location was confirmed angiographically. Advancement of the laser catheter through the lesion was performed during 10–30 s of energy delivery, dependent on lesion morphology and length of lesion. During this procedure only gentle pressure was applied on the device. The procedure was repeated at least twice and after each irradiation cycle control angiography was performed. The intervention was terminated if no visible improvement in luminal diameter was observed. Angiography of the target vessel was repeated after a control period of 5, 10, 15, and 20 min to confirm lesion morphology after intervention. Due to the results of coronary excimer laser angioplasty in our first series the protocol of laser angioplasty was modified in the second and third series of patients: 1) The total irradiation time of the lesion was sought to be limited up to 100 s in an attempt to reduce vessel wall irritation due to photoacoustic and mechanical effects; 2) Irradiation cycle length was 3 s with a 2-s interval between two cycles to reduce additional vessel damage by heat and gas generation; 3) Additional balloon dilatation was performed in those patients only, in whom a lesion of > 50% was still present or if vessel occlusion occurred after laser ablation.

Table 2. Patient population (second series).

		(n)
Total		40
Gender	M	31
	F	9
Mean age (years)		57 ± 9
Extent CAD	1-VD	24
	2-VD	12
	3-VD	4
Target vessel	LAD	28
	CIRC	3
	RCA	9
Lesion morphology		
-eccentric		24
-concentric		9
-occlusion		3
-long segmental		4
Lesion length		
>10 mm		6
<10 mm		34
CCS	1	2
	2	18
	3	17
	4	3

(Abbreviations same as Table 1)

If catheter exchange was necessary, the original guide wire was connected to an extension wire and the primarily used catheter was pulled back, leaving the guide wire in the periphery of the target vessel. Subsequent balloon dilatation was performed using a monorail balloon (RX, ACS, Santa Ana, California).

All patients were monitored in the coronary care unit for at least 24 h after intervention. Blood samples for enzyme levels of CK and CKMB were taken every 3 h. Twelve-lead electrocardiograms were carried out every 6 h; 12 to 36 h after the intervention, early follow-up angiography was performed.

During the time of follow-up 47/26/34 patients of series 1, 2, and 3, respectively, underwent follow-up angiography after intervention.

Qualitative and quantitative angiographic analysis

Two experienced cardiologists made a qualitative analysis of the coronary angiograms before, during, and after intervention, and at the early follow-up and late follow-up angiography. Additionally, all films were analyzed using quantitative arteriographic techniques. The length of the lesion, minimal stenosis diameter, and percent stenosis were calculated. Success of laser angioplasty and balloon dilatation was defined as a

114

Table 3. Patient population (third series).

		(n)
Total		47 (48 interventions)
Gender	M	43
	F	4
Mean age (years)		56 ± 8
Extent CAD	1-VD	27
	2-VD	12
	3-VD	8
Target vessel	LAD	31
	CIRC	3
	RCA	14
Lesion morphology		
-eccentric		32
-concentric		10
-occlusion		2
-long segmental		5
Lesion length		
>10 mm		10
<10 mm		38
CCS	1	4
	2	25
	3	15
	4	3

(Abbreviations same as Table 1)

reduction of lesion severity to less than 50% from pre- to post intervention and early follow-up angiography.

For all patients restenosis was defined as a loss of at least 50% of the gain in luminal diameter achieved at angioplasty (NHLBI IV).

Results

First series

In five of 60 patients it was not possible to place the catheter in an axial position within the vessel [1] or to pass the lesion with the guide wire [4], and, thus, laser irradiation was not performed in order to avoid vessel injury (see Table 4). The results of this series have been published in detail [11].

In 55 patients in whom laser angioplasty was possible, percent stenosis decreased from 81 ± 17% before, to 37 ± 17% after laser treatment. In 23 of these 55 patients (42%), no additional balloon angioplasty was performed. In 32 patients, percent stenosis decreased from 85 ± 14% before, to 44 ± 14% after coronary excimer laser treatment, and conventional balloon dilatation had to be carried out, resulting in a residual percent stenosis of 24 ± 15%.

115

Table 4. First series: Coronary excimer laser angioplasty.

n: 60

Lesion not passed   n: 5

Stable AP   n: 4
Unstable AP   n: 1

Ablation performed n: 55

Stable angina pectoris n: 45

Unstable angina pectoris n: 10

Successful laser ablation n: 21

Vessel closure after ablation n: 7

Successful PTCA n: 7

Incomplete result after laser ablation n: 17

Successful PTCA n: 17

Successful laser ablation n: 2

Vessel closure after ablation n: 4

Early death n: 1

Myocardial infarction n: 2

Successful PTCA n: 1

Incomplete results after laser ablation n: 4

Successful PTCA n: 4

116

Coronary occlusion after laser angioplasty occurred within 10 min in 11 patients and was treated with balloon angioplasty. Intracoronary nitroglycerin failed to relieve vessel closure in all cases. Two patients, in whom the occluded vessel could not be reopened, developed Q-wave infarctions with a rise in creatine kinase and MB isoenzyme creatine kinase values.

Angiographic evidence of intracoronary thrombi was seen in seven patients. Dissections within the area of ablation were documented in 11 patients. In 19 patients vasospasm was reversible by intracoronary nitroglycerin or nifedipine. Perforations did not occur.

In a subgroup of 10 patients with unstable angina pectoris, laser irradiation of the ischemia-related lesion was successful in only two patients. In the remaining eight patients, additional balloon angioplasty was necessary due to acute vessel closure and due to an incomplete result in four patients, respectively. In five of these eight patients, additional balloon dilatation was successful, and the following clinical course was unremarkable. However, one patient of this group died soon after the intervention and two patients experienced a myocardial infarction. Thus, all serious complications occurred in patients with unstable angina in this series (see Table 4).

During a 6-month follow-up period no patient died. Myocardial infarction did not occur in the control period. In 47 patients late follow-up angiography was performed. Five patients refused late follow-up angiography. All five patients had no episodes of chest pain and no signs of ischemia during treadmill excercise at maximum work load. In 22 patients the quantitative analysis of the target lesion revealed a restenosis. In six of these 22 patients an occlusion was found at late follow-up angiography. Reintervention by balloon dilatation or aortocoronary bypass grafting was performed in 15 patients. In our first series the incidence of reintervention as well as the incidence of restenosis was higher in those patients, who were initially treated with laser and balloon angioplasty than in those patients, who were treated with laser therapy alone (see Table 7).

Second series

In five of 40 patients laser angioplasty was not performed, because the laser catheter could not be positioned to the stenosis coaxially (two patients) or vessel occlusion of the target vessel was present and the guide wire could not be passed across the lesion, (three patients; see Table 5).

No additional balloon angioplasty was performed in 24 of the 35 patients in whom laser angioplasty was possible. Percent stenosis decreased from $74 \pm 13\%$ before to $31 \pm 14\%$ after laser angioplasty. In 11 patients additional balloon dilatation was performed after laser ablation. Conventional balloon angioplasty was performed in five patients due to vessel occlusion, and in six patients because the angiographic result was not thought to be sufficient. In these patients percent stenosis decreased from $69 \pm 11\%$ at preintervention to $20 \pm 15\%$ after combined laser and balloon dilatation.

Coronary occlusion after laser ablation occurred in six of the 35 patients. Occlusion occurred within 15 min after laser irradiation, although the initial angiographic results were sufficient, with a residual minimal lumen diameter of 1.51 ± 1.43 mm. In two of the six patients intraluminal lucencies suggestive of intraluminal thrombi were seen which were no longer detectable after subsequent balloon angioplasty. In five of the six patients balloon dilatation was successful and persistent patency of the target vessel

Table 5. Second series: Coronary excimer laser angioplasty.

Results

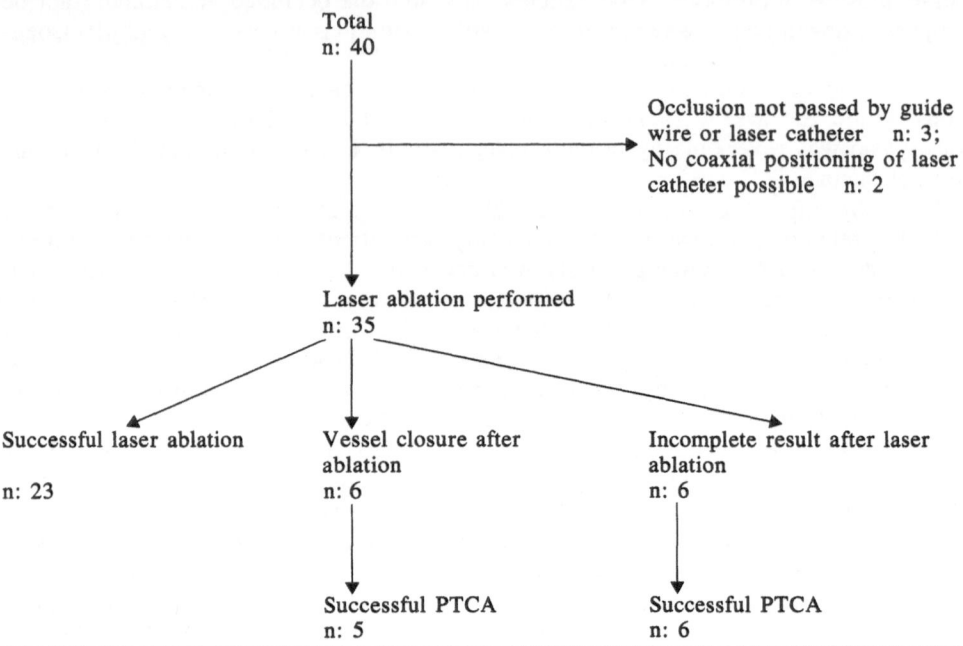

Total
n: 40

Occlusion not passed by guide
wire or laser catheter   n: 3;
No coaxial positioning of laser
catheter possible   n: 2

Laser ablation performed
n: 35

Successful laser ablation

n: 23

Vessel closure after
ablation
n: 6

Incomplete result after laser
ablation
n: 6

Successful PTCA
n: 5

Successful PTCA
n: 6

Table 6. Third series: Coronary excimer laser angioplasty.

Results

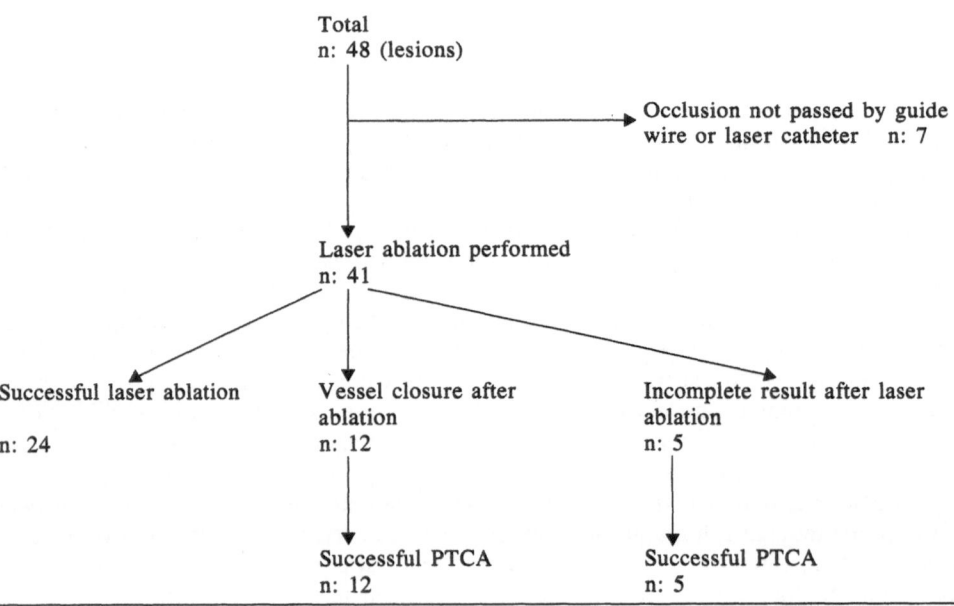

Total
n: 48 (lesions)

Occlusion not passed by guide
wire or laser catheter   n: 7

Laser ablation performed
n: 41

Successful laser ablation

n: 24

Vessel closure after
ablation
n: 12

Incomplete result after laser
ablation
n: 5

Successful PTCA
n: 12

Successful PTCA
n: 5

Table 7. Summary of incidence of restenosis within the 6-month follow up period (first series).

	Total group (n)	Laser ablation only (n)	Laser ablation and balloon angioplasty (n)
Late follow-up angiography	47	19	28
Restenosis	22	6	16
Reintervention	15	5	10
PTCA	12	4	8
Coronary artery bypass graft	3	1	2

could be achieved. One patient, in whom the vessel could not be reopened, developed a Q-wave infarction in the perfusion area of the target vessel with a typical rise of CK and CKMB. After discharge from the coronary care unit this patient died 48 h after intervention. One patient with a complete occlusion was successfully treated with additional laser irradiation and left the catheterization laboratory with a patent vessel.

One perforation occurred in a patient with a 90% proximal and eccentric left anterior descending artery lesion. Due to severe vasospasms, thrombus formation and early occlusion of the target vessel balloon angioplasty was performed, thus restoring antegrade flow. Immediately after PTCA, extravasation of dye was terminated. The 24-h control angiogram documented a sufficient angiographic result without signs of dye extravasation. No pericardial effusion was present immediately after intervention or during follow-up.

At the 24-h control angiogram in two patients, occlusions were found which were successfully dilated the same day. Neither patient developed a rise of CK and CKMB nor had electrocardiographic changes indicative of myocardial infarction. During the 6-month follow-up period, one patient died 4 months after intervention while playing tennis. According to his family physician, he had complained about symptoms of angina pectoris prior to his death; an autopsy could not be carried out. Myocardial infarction did not occur within the control period. The individual data of the 26 patients in whom late follow-up angiography was performed are provided in Table 8. In 12 patients, quantitative analysis of the target lesion revealed a restenosis according to the applied criteria. Reintervention of either balloon dilatation or laser angioplasty was performed in all 12 patients; five patients refused the control angiogram. None of these patients had episodes of chest pain and none had signs of ischemia during treadmill excercise at maximum work load.

Third series

Coronary excimer laser angioplasty could not be carried out in seven of 48 patients, because of failure of guidewire placement [3] or placement or passage of the laser catheter [4] (see Table 6).

In 40 patients in whom laser angioplasty could be performed, percent stenosis decreased from $70 \pm 8\%$ before, to $38 \pm 14\%$ after laser treatment. In 17 patients additional balloon dilatation was performed due to acute vessel closure in 12 patients, and

119

Table 8. Summary of incidence of restenosis within the 6-month follow up period (second series).

	Total group (n)	Laser ablation only (n)	Laser ablation and balloon angioplasty (n)
Late follow-up angiography	26	17	9
Restenosis	12	8	4
Reintervention	12	8	4
PTCA	10	7	3
Coronary artery bypass graft	2	1	1

Table 9. Summary of incidence of restenosis within the 6-month follow up period (third series).

	Total group (n)	Laser ablation only (n)	Laser ablation and balloon angioplasty (n)
Late follow-up angiography	34	20	14
Restenosis	11	8	3
Reintervention	9	7	2
PTCA	9	7	2
Coronary artery bypass graft	0	0	0

due to an unsufficient angiographic result in five patients. In these 17 patients percent stenosis decreased from $70 \pm 9\%$ to $42 \pm 15\%$ after laser angioplasty to $29 \pm 14\%$ after subsequent balloon dilatation. Coronary occlusion after laser treatment occurred within 20 min in 12 of the 40 patients. In all 12 patients subsequent balloon dilatation could be performed successfully, resulting in persistent patency of the target vessel. There was no perforation, myocardial infarction, death or early occlusion in this series of patients.

During the time of follow-up there was one late death and no myocardial infarction. Late follow-up angiography was performed in 34 patients of this series (see Table 9). Five patients refused late follow-up angiography. Four of these patients had no episodes of angina pectoris and no signs of ischemia during treadmill excercise at maximum work load. According to the applied criteria, a restenosis was found in 11 patients. Reintervention was carried out in nine patients. All patients in whom a reintervention was performed were treated with balloon dilatation. Seven of these patients were initially treated with laser angioplasty alone, and two patients were treated with a combination of laser and balloon treatment.

Discussion

PTCA was initially reserved for patients with single-vessel disease who had a single, concentric, subtotal stenosis, good left-ventricular function, and stable but medically refractory angina [5, 8]. Although these candidates still remain ideal candidates for

PTCA, they account for only a minority of those patients who currently undergo balloon dilatation. The exponential growth of PTCA is the result of changing criteria for selection of patients, improved technology, growing operator experience, and the number of patients who have restenosis and require repeat dilatation [8].

Major changes in the technology of PTCA equipment have occurred since its introduction in 1977. These changes have faciliated the expanded use of dilatation and the improvement in the success rate of approximately 60% in 1977, to 90% in 1988 [5, 9]. However, the rate of restenotic lesions following balloon dilatation seems to be unaffected. In published series, restenosis rates have averaged 30%, predominantly in patients with single-vessel disease. In patients with multivessel dilatation, restenosis rates are higher [4, 7, 12, 13, 15, 16]. As already alluded to, a decrease of restenosis rates may be expected if plaque removal rather than plaque remodeling is performed, which may go along with a reduction of vessel wall injury. Besides the crucial issue of restenosis, the success of PTCA is limited in bifurcational lesions, calcified hard lesions with elastic recoil and distal vessel disease. It might be speculated that patients with coronary artery disease and these types of lesions may preferably be treated with laser angioplasty, which actually results in tissue removal. This method might be of special interest in reducing the probability of side branch occlusions in bifurcations and enhancing plaque reduction in hard atherosclerotic tissue.

The early trials of coronary excimer laser angioplasty demonstrated the feasibility and safety of this technique as an alternative to PTCA in the treatment of patients with coronary artery disease [10, 11, 14, 17, 19]. Since every new method has to be compared with the current gold standards, it has to be stated that the efficacy of excimer treatment alone is still reduced in comparison with PTCA, although considerable improvement is documented in our second and third series of patients.

The progress achieved by new catheter devices with greater variability, higher flexibility, and improved energy transmission is reflected in an increase of successful stand-alone laser angioplasty from 38% in our first, to more than 60% in our second and third series of patients. Larger catheter diameters definitely result in larger lumen diameters and reduce the need for additional balloon angioplasty. Additionally, improved energy transmission improves ablative properties and enhances the efficacy of plaque removal. This results in a reduction of mechanical vessel wall trauma and shortens treatment time.

However, it should be taken into consideration that several other factors may have contributed to the improved success rate. With growing operator experience the procedure was modified: 1) irradiation time was shortened, 2) larger laser catheters were used following laser irradiation with smaller diameter catheter devices, if the angiographic result was not sufficient, and 3) additional balloon angioplasty was only performed in those patients with occlusion after laser ablation or with a residual stenosis >50% after a 20-min control period. Secondly, all patients of the second and third series were selected in regard to their clinical status and their coronary morphology. Due to the unfavorable results of coronary excimer laser angioplasty in patients with unstable angina pectoris, unstable patients were excluded in the second and third series. Additionally, laser irradiation was not attempted in severe vessel tortuosities of the target vessel. It remains open to question if further procedural modifications and the application of even larger catheter systems may help to improve primary success rates.

The incidence of acute coronary occlusions following laser angioplasty is approximately 20% and is comparable in all series of patients. Coronary occlusions constitute a major cause for the need of additional balloon angioplasty and are the major cause

121

for acute myocardial infarction. The only acute death in our study group occurred in a 71-year-old unstable patient with triple-vessel disease, in whom severe vasospasms and vessel occlusion followed laser treatment in a proximal left anterior descending artery. The reason for early vessel occlusion following laser irradiation remains largely unknown. Although all patients received intracoronary nitroglycerin before the procedure and additional intracoronary nitroglycerin and nifedipine if occlusion occurred, underlying coronary spasm may still be of outstanding importance for vessel occlusion. However, it is conceivable that spasm might not be the only mechanism involved, and that dissection and thrombosis, although not often seen angiographically, may be a second major reason for occlusion [2, 18].

The overall incidence of restenosis in the first, second, and third series was, with 40%, 34%, and 28%, decreasing. Concluding from the summarized results of restenosis from all three series it, therefore, cannot yet be answered if coronary excimer laser angioplasty improves the long-term success rates in comparison to balloon dilatation. A larger number of patients will be necessary to detect statistically significant differences between patients treated with either balloon or excimer laser angioplasty.

Clinical implications

Coronary excimer laser angioplasty is safe and effective in ablating atherosclerotic plaque in patients with coronary artery disease. The need for additional balloon angioplasty due to vessel occlusion or due to an insuffecent angiographic result is decreasing as a result of the application of improved transmission devices. However, the efficacy of excimer laser angioplasty in the native coronary circulation is still reduced in comparison to conventional balloon dilatation. It is, therefore, necessary to improve laser light sources and catheter technology before randomized clinical trials are conducted which will have to define potentially primary indications, as well as the rate of restenosis for coronary excimer laser angioplasty.

References

1. Badimon L, Badimon JJ, Galvez A, Chesebro JH, Fuster V (1986) Influence of arterial damage and wall shear rate on platelet deposition. Arteriosclerosis 6: 312–320
2. Baumbach A, Haase KK, Voelker W, Mauser M, Karsch KR (1991) Effects of intracoronary nitroglycerin on lumen diameter during early follow-up angiography after coronary excimer laser atherectomy. Eur Heart J (in press)
3. (1980) Editorial: Why the American decline in coronary heart disease? Lancet 1: 183
4. Grigg LE, Kay TW, Valentine PA, Larkins R, Flower DJ, Manolas EG, O'Dea K, Sinclair AJ, Hopper JL, Hunt D (1989) Determinants of restenosis and lack of effect of dieatry supplementation with eicosapentaenoic acid on the incidence of coronary artery restenosis after angioplasty. J Am Coll Cardiol 13: 665–672
5. Grüntzig AR, Senning A, Siegenthaler WE (1979) Nonoperative dilatation of coronary artery stenosis: percutaneous transluminal coronary angioplasty. N Engl J Med 301: 61–68
6. Hanke H, Oberhoff M, Strohschneider T, Betz E, Karsch KR (1990) Time course of intimal and medial smooth muscle cell proliferation following experimental angioplasty. Circ Res 67: 651–659
7. Holmes DR Jr, Vlietstra RE, Smith HC, Vetrovec GW, Kent KM, Cowley MJ, Faxon DP, Gruentzig AR, Kelsey SF, Detre KM, Van Raden MJ, Mock MB (1984) Restenosis after percutaneous transluminal coronary angioplasty (PTCA): a report from the PTCA Registry of the National Heart, Lung and Blood Institute. Am J Cardiol 53: 77C–81C

8. Holmes DR Jr, Vlietstra RE (1989) Balloon angioplasty in acute and chronic coronary artery disease. JAMA 261: 2109–2115
9. Holmes DR, Vlietstra RE, Reiter SJ, Bresnahan DR (1990) Advances in interventional cardiology. Mayo Clin Proc 65: 565–583
10. Karsch KR, Haase KK, Mauser M, Ickrath O, Voelker W, Duda S, Seipel L (1989) Percutaneous coronary excimer laser angioplasty: Initial clinical results. Lancet 2: 647–650
11. Karsch KR, Haase KK, Voelker W, Baumbach A, Mauser M, Seipel L (1990) Percutaneous coronary excimer laser angioplasty in patients with stable and unstable angina pectoris. Circulation 81: 1849–1859
12. Kent KM, Bentivoglio LG, Block PC, Bourassa MG, Cowley MJ, Dorros G, Detre KM, Gosselin AJ, Gruentzig AR, Kelsey SF, Mock MB, Mullin SM, Passamani ER, Myler RK, Simpson J, Stertzer SH, Van Raden MJ, Williams DO (1984) Long-term efficacy of percutaneous transluminal coronary angioplasty (PTCA): report from the National Heart, Lung, and Blood Institute PTCA Registry. Am J Cardiol 53: 27C–31C
13. Leimgruber PP, Roubin GS, Hollman J, Cotsonis GA, Meier B, Douglas JS, King SB III, Gruentzig AR (1986) Restenosis after successful corornary angioplasty in patients with single-vessel disease. Circulation 73: 710–717
14. Litvack F, Margolis J, Rothbaum D, Kent K, Breshnahan J, Unterecker W, Cummins F, Forrester J and the ELCA investigators (1990) Excimer laser coronary angioplasty – acute results of the first 685 consecutive patients. Circulation 82: III–71 (abstract)
15. Liu MW, Roubin GS, King SB III (1989) Restenosis after coronary angioplasty: Potential biological determinants and role of intimal hyperplasia. Circulation 79: 1374–1387
16. Roubin G, Redd D, Leimgruber P, et al. (1986) Restenosis after multilesion and multivessel coronary angioplasty. J Am Coll Cardiol 7: II–20 (abstract)
17. Sanborn T, Hershman R, Torre S, Sherman W, Cohen M, Ambrose JA (1989) Percutaneous excimer laser coronary angioplasty. Lancet 2: 616: letter
18. Steg PG, Rongione AJ, Gal D, De Jesus S, Clarke RH, Isner JM (1989) Pulsed ultraviolet laser irradiation produces endothelium-independent relaxation of vascular smooth muscle. Circulation 79: 189–197
19. Werner GS, Buchwald A, Unterberg C, Voth E, Kreuzer H, Wiegand V (1990) Recanalization of chronic coronary occlusions by excimer-laser angioplasty. J Am Coll Cardiol 15: 245 (abstract)

Authors's address:
K. K. Haase
Division of Cardiology
Medical Clinic III
Otfried Müllerstr. 10
7400 Tübingen, FRG

Holmium: YAG Coronary Laser Angioplasty (HOLCA). The American Experience

C. J. White, S. R. Ramee

Section on Cardiology, Department of Internal Medicine, Ochsner Medical Institutions, New Orleans, Louisiana, USA

Introduction

The development of a clinically effective laser angioplasty system for the percutaneous recanalization of occlusive coronary artery atherosclerosis is a complex task involving the selection of an optimal laser wavelength and coupling this energy source to a delivery catheter which can safely and effectively recanalize lesions in the coronary arteries. The *potential* advantages of using laser energy for percutaneous revascularization of coronary artery disease include; 1) reducing the restenosis rate that occurs following balloon angioplasty in approximately one-third of patients [5, 8]; 2) reducing the frequency of abrupt artery occlusion and emergency coronary bypass grafting associated with balloon angioplasty [1]; and 3) extending the indications for percutaneous recanalization to patients currently considered to be poor candidates for balloon angioplasty, such as those with unfavorable lesions or diffuse disease [12, 15].

In selecting an ideal laser energy source for recanalization there are several important criteria that must be met. First, the laser should be mechanically reliable and easy for the physician to operate. Lasers which require the presence of an one-site laser engineer for frequent adjustments to the laser or frequent alignment of the internal optics are not acceptable for general clinical use. The laser beam should be easily and efficiently coupled to optical delivery fibers ranging in diameter from 50 μm to 200 μm. Ideally the laser should be pulsed [11] and the wavelength highly absorbed by the target tissue to increase the precision of ablation and avoid unwarranted effects on surrounding tissues [2, 4, 10, 11, 14, 16–18].

The holmium: YAG laser, a near-infrared laser with a primary wavelength at 2.1 μm, satisfies the above criteria for an ideal laser. Vascular tissue and atherosclerotic plaque contain a large amount of water which serves as a very effective absorber for several near-infrared laser wavelengths including holmium: YAG (2.1 μm) and erbium: YAG (2.9 μm) (Fig. 1). The closer the peak of the laser wavelength is to the absorbtion peak of water in this case, the more efficient the energy absorption, the shallower the penetration, and the less energy will be needed to ablate tissue (Table 1) [3].

The holmium: YAG laser is a solid-state laser which greatly simplifies its daily use and minimizes the need for frequent adjustments and maintenance. The holmium: YAG laser beam is easily coupled to small diameter silica fibers which are not available for the erbium: YAG wavelength.

The holmium: YAG laser is a pulsed laser and can be operated in a free-running mode with microsecond pulses or in the Q-switched mode with nanosecond pulses [7].

125

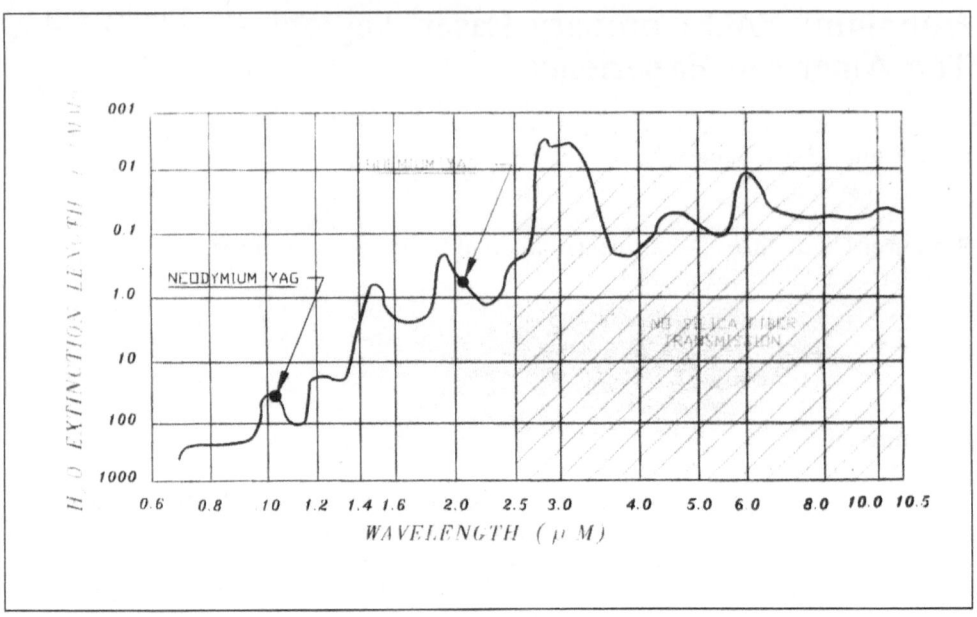

Fig. 1. Chart depicting water absorption vs laser wavelength. Note that silica fibers will not transmit light above 2.5 μm in wavelength.

Table 1. Comparison of tissue absorption parameters for near-infrared lasers.

Laser	Wavelength (μm)	α (Tissue) (cm^{-1})	Penetration depth (μm)
Erbium: YAG	2.94	10,000	1
Holmium: YAG	2.06	35	286
Neodymium: YAG	1.06	4	2,500

The absorption coefficients (α) assume a tissue water content of 60% (Adapted from [3]).

One advantage in using pulsed lasers is that, as long as there is time between pulses for the tissue to cool to the baseline temperature (thermal relaxation time), there will be minimal thermal effects associated with the ablation.

The purpose of this study was to determine the feasibilty and safety of a holmium: YAG laser angioplasty system including two multifiber delivery catheters for the percutaneous recanalization of coronary artery lesions. This trial, which is ongoing, is not intended as a test of the efficacy of laser angioplasty alone, owing to the relatively small diameters of the multifiber catheters. We recognized in designing the trial that concomitant treatment with adjunctive angioplasty devices would be needed to successfully complete the procedures in a majority of patients.

126

Methods

Patient selection

Patients were considered candidates for this experimental coronary laser angioplasty trial if they had evidence of coronary ischemia such as symptom-limiting stable angina pectoris, a positive exercise study for coronary ischemia, or unstable angina pectoris. The patients were required to have coronary artery lesion(s) suitable for elective PTCA and the ability to give informed consent. This protocol was approved by the Food and Drug Administration (USA) and our hospital institutional review board's Clinical Investigation Committee.

At present, seven lesions have been treated in the six patients that were entered in this trial, and their demographic data are shown in Table 2. The mean age of the six patients was 58.1 years with a range from 38 to 69 years. There were five males and one female. Three of the patients had unstable angina defined as angina at rest, and three patients had stable angina following myocardial infarction. Patient number two had undergone prior coronary artery bypass surgery, and laser angioplasty was performed in a saphenous vein graft to the right coronary artery. Patient number five had two sequential lesions in the proximal and middle left anterior descending artery which were both treated with the laser.

Laser angioplasty

The patients were pretreated with oral aspirin, 325 mg per day, and a calcium channel blocker, usually diltiazem. Femoral artery percutaneous access was obtained using the modified Seldinger technique and a 9F arterial sheath with a hemostatic valve (USCI, Billerica, Massachusetts, USA) was inserted. Ten thousand units of heparin were administered and a 9F coronary angioplasty guiding catheter (Medtronic, Minneapolis, Minnesota, USA) was advanced to the coronary ostium. Baseline angiography of the lesion to be treated was performed in two orthogonal views and 200 µg of intracoronary nitroglycerin were administered prior to laser angioplasty.

The holmium: YAG (2.1 µm) laser system (Trimedyne, Tustin, California) was used in the free-running mode with a 250-µsec pulsewidth (full width at half-maximum) at

Table 2. Patient demographic data.

Patient No.	Age	Sex	Risk factors	Clinical symptom
1.	56	M	HTN	UA
2.	69	M	DM, CHOL	UA
3.	60	F	HTN, CHOL	UA
4.	62	M	HTN, CHOL	SA, MI
5.	61	M	TOB	SA, MI
6.	38	M	TOB, CHOL	SA, MI

M=male, F=female, HTN=hypertension, DM=diabetes mellitus, CHOL=hypercholesterolemia, TOB=tobacco use, UA=unstable angina, SA=stable angina, MI=prior myocardial infarction.

5 Hz. The laser delivered 200 to 400 mJ/pulse measured in air with a power meter. A 0.014-inch angioplasty guidewire (High-Torque Floppy, ACS, Santa Clara, California) was advanced across the lesion to be treated, and the laser delivery catheter was advanced to the lesion over the guidewire.

We delivered the laser energy through either a 1.6-mm or 2.0-mm diameter multifiber catheter (Trimedyne, Tustin, California) which accepted a 0.014-inch angioplasty guidewire (ACS, Santa Clara, California) through its central lumen (Fig. 2). The 1.6-mm diameter catheter contained 19 fibers, each of which is 100 μm in diameter and delivered fluences of 335 mJ/mm^2 to 2,680 mJ/mm^2, and the 2.0 mm diameter catheter contained 28 fibers arranged circumferentially around a central guidewire lumen and delivered fluences ranging from 219 mJ/mm^2 to 1,754 mJ/mm^2.

We began each laser treatment at approximately 200 mJ/pulse and delivered the energy in 2-s to 5-s bursts, with very gentle pressure on the catheter to maintain contact with the lesion. If the catheter would not advance, the laser energy delivery was increased in increments of approximately 50 mJ/pulse to a maximum of 400 mJ/pulse. Very gentle pressure was applied to the laser catheter when crossing the lesions, and at no point was the catheter forced across a lesion. It was our goal to allow the laser to cross the lesion as a result of tissue ablation rather than by performing a mechanical dilation.

Following laser angioplasty, the patient was observed for 15 min and angiography of the treated stenosis was performed. If the stenosis had not been reduced to less than a 20% residual stenosis, the operator was free to choose an adjunctive method to further reduce the post-laser stenosis. The angiograms were reviewed and diameter stenosis was calculated using calipers, comparing the lesions with the nearest proximal segment of the artery that was considered to be of normal diameter.

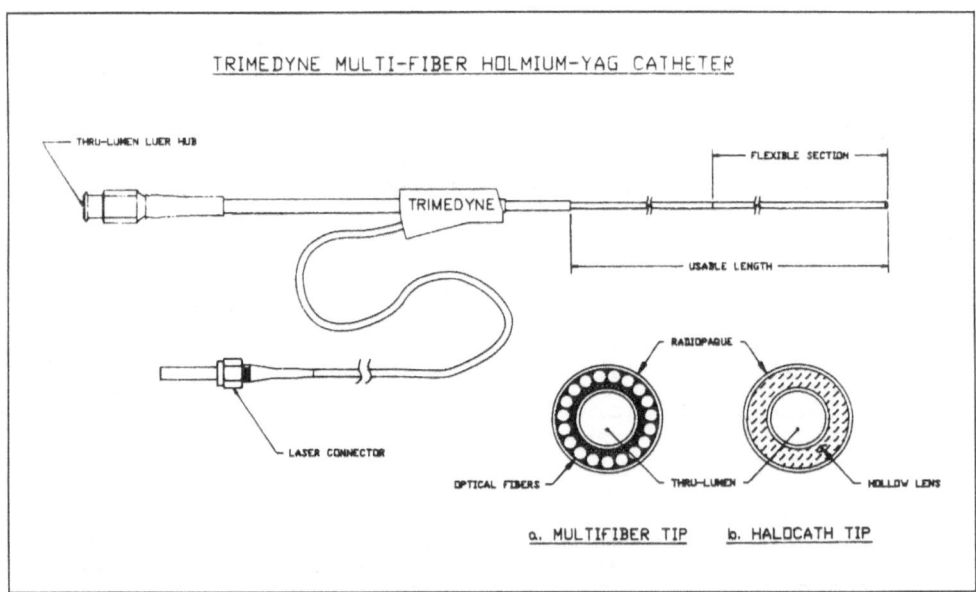

Fig. 2. Schematic drawing of the multifiber catheter. Two tips are shown: a) the multifiber tip, and b) a lensed tip called the "halocath".

Statistics

Continous variables were compared using Student's *t*-test for paired data. A p value ≤ 0.05 was considered as a significant difference. Other values are shown as the mean ± the standard deviation where appropriate.

Results

Successful delivery of holium: YAG laser energy and partial recanalization of the coronary stenoses was accomplished in all seven lesions attempted (Table 3). No densely calcified lesions were seen on fluoroscopy in this small group of patients. The mean length of the lesions attempted was 15.9 ± 7.9 mm (mean ± SD) with a range of 5 to 25 mm. The mean maximal energy delivered was 314.3 ± 80 mJ/pulse with a range from 200 to 400 mJ/pulse. The total energy required to cross the lesions was 12.0 ± 4.3 Joules with a range of 7 to 21 Joules.

The baseline coronary stenosis averaged $96.6 \pm 3.5\%$ (mean ± SD) which was reduced to $38.6 \pm 24.1\%$ (p = 0.0006) after laser angioplasty (Fig. 3). One patient with a 99% stenosis in a 2.5 mm artery was treated with laser alone and was left with a residual stenosis of 10%. Following laser therapy, balloon angioplasty was used in two lesions and atherectomy (Simpson Atherocath, Peripheral Systems Group, Santa Clara, California) was used in the four remaining lesions to reduce the final mean stenosis to $12.9 \pm 4.9\%$ (Fig. 4).

There were no complications associated with laser energy delivery. The patients did not report any sensations other than intermittent angina pectoris during laser treatment, presumably due to temporary occlusion of the artery when the laser catheter was engaged. No large dissections, coronary spasm, or emboli were identified on angiograms following laser recanalization. One patient underwent coronary angioscopy following laser treatment, revealing evidence of numerous superficial intimal tears at the site of the lesion. There was no evidence of tissue charring, but the walls of the neolumen had a dull red appearance consistent with tissue removal by laser ablation. Four patients had tissue specimens removed via the atherectomy catheter. The samples showed no evidence of thermal charring, but there was evidence of thermal tissue effect.

Two patients (Nos. 1 and 6) had abrupt occlusion of the treated artery immediately following coronary atherectomy. There was no suggestion of impending artery occlu-

Table 3. Results by lesion following laser angioplasty.

Lesion	Artery	Length (mm)	Maximum energy (mJ/Pulse)	Total energy (J)	Adjunctive device
1	LCX	24	350	7.0	Atherectomy (3.5 mm)
2	SVG	10	200	11.0	Balloon (3.5 mm)
3	LAD	5	200	12.0	Balloon (3.0 mm)
4	RCA	25	400	12.0	None
5	LAD	10	350	10.5	Atherectomy (3.0 mm)
6	LAD	22	350	10.5	Atherectomy (3.0 mm)
7	LAD	15	350	21.0	Atherectomy (3.0 mm)

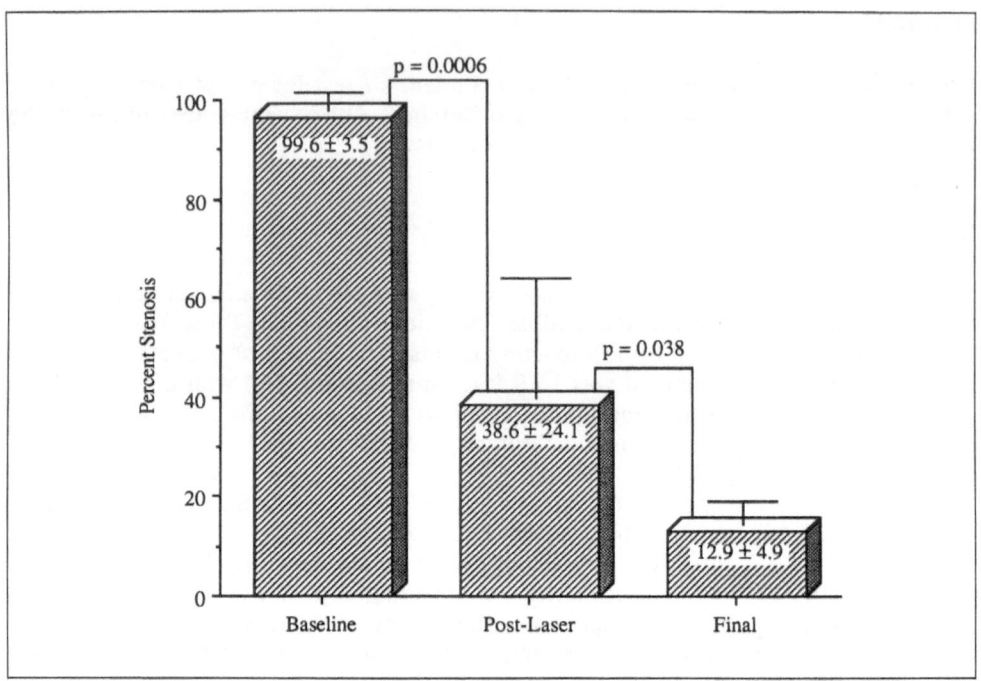

Fig. 3. Bar graph showing the percent luminal stenosis (mean ± standard deviation) at baseline, post-laser, and following adjunctive therapy.

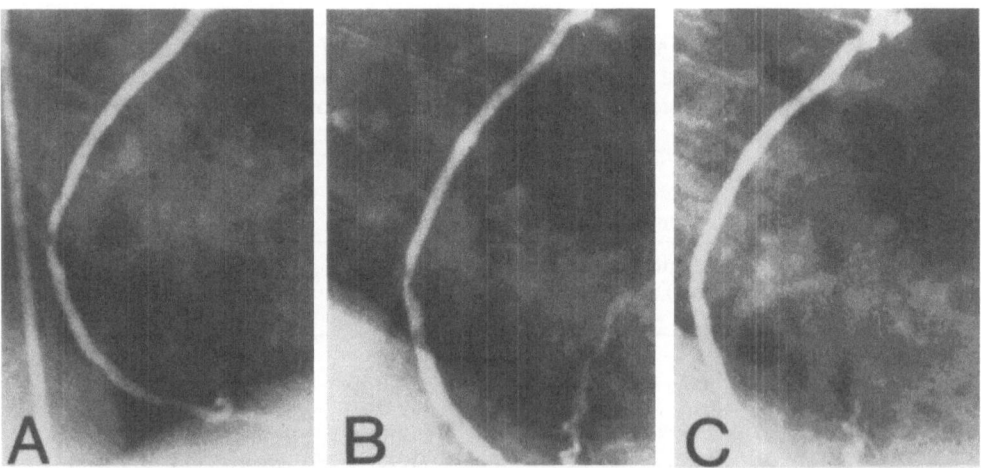

Fig. 4. A) Baseline angiography of a saphenous vein bypass graft. B) Mild residual stenosis following passage of a 2.0 mm multifiber catheter. C) Final result after 4.0 mm balloon dilation.

sion on angiography after laser therapy alone. The occlusions were treated by repeat atherectomy and intracoronary thrombolytic therapy with urokinase and an excellent final angiographic result was obtained in both patients without evidence of myocardial damage. Patient No. 6 subsequently occluded the treated artery again several hours after the initial procedure and multiple attempts to restore patency of the artery failed. The patient received an intracoronary stent which succeeded in restoring patency, but the patient had electrocardiographic and enzymatic evidence of a myocardial infarction.

Discussion

In this very small initial series of patients, we have found that the use of a holmium: YAG laser with a multifiber delivery catheter appears both feasible and safe. A significant reduction in the luminal diameter stenosis was achieved with the laser alone, reducing the mean stenosis to less than 50% in five of the seven lesions treated, however, we chose to further optimize the result with adjunctive angioplasty therapy in six of the seven lesions.

The question of whether the predominant effect of the laser catheters is, in fact, tissue ablation or merely mechanical dilation of the lesion by crossing with the catheter remains. In one patient, we used angioscopy to directly view the treated lesion and observed a qualitative improvement in the luminal diameter without evidence of thermal charring. We also obtained tissue samples with the atherectomy catheter following laser ablation which confirmed a tissue effect of the laser without thermal charring. Further support for tissue ablation as the mechanism for improving the luminal diameter is that the minimum fluence delivered by the multifiber catheters (219 mJ/mm^2) was above the threshold required for ablation of non-calcified human atherosclerotic aorta tissue (160 mJ/mm^2) for the holmium: YAG laser in the free-running mode as reported by Kopchock et al. [7].

Two of our patients experienced abrupt occlusion of the treated artery after adjunctive therapy with coronary atherectomy. It is impossible to know to what extent the laser treatment contributed to this complication. We saw no evidence of impending artery occlusion in these patients following laser angioplasty alone, and artery occlusion is a known complication of atherectomy. Larger numbers of patients will need to be studied, and hopefully more patients can be treated with laser recanalization alone as larger multifiber catheters become available.

The multifiber laser catheters used in this study were prototype devices which will require improvement in the future. The distal tip of the catheter is relatively rigid and could be made more flexible to facilitate the catheter's ability to track over the angioplasty guidewire and remain in a concentric position with the lumen of the artery. Modifications to decrease the "dead space" between the laser fibers and the catheter, as well as improvement in the catheter's performance, including both trackability and pushability are needed.

For coronary laser angioplasty to succeed as a viable clinical technique, it must stand alone as a percutaneous recanalization device and not rely on adjunctive balloon angioplasty to complete the procedure. One of the limitations of current laser angioplasty delivery systems is the small diameter neolumens, approximately 1.0 mm to 2.2 mm, created with current multifiber laser angioplasty catheters [6, 9, 13]. The average diameter of coronary arteries currently approached with balloon angioplasty is much nearer to 3.0 mm, therefore a stand-alone coronary laser system should be designed to create recanalized lumens of 2.5 mm to 3.5 mm in diameter.

The current limitation in the diameter of recanalized lumens with laser angioplasty systems is determined by the inner lumen of coronary guiding catheters through which the laser catheter must pass to reach the coronary artery. At present, 8F and 9F guiding catheters will accept a maximum diameter catheter of 2.0 mm to 2.2 mm, which is the current maximum size of the neolumen created with multifiber catheters.

One method by which small diameter catheters may be used to create larger lumens is to attach a diverging lens on the distal end of the laser catheter to increase the "spot size" irradiated by the laser, and thereby increase the size of the channel created by laser ablation. This increase in the area irradiated by the laser markedly increases the energy necessary for ablation of the larger volume of target tissue. Current excimer laser systems operate with a relatively narrow margin with energy delivery slightly above the threshold for tissue ablation, but below the damage threshold of the silica fibers, which makes it unlikely that excimer systems can take advantage of a diverging lens to increase the size of the neolumen. The holmium: YAG laser, however, is efficiently transmitted through silica fibers, and can easily generate an energy density sufficient to allow a diverging lens to be used [19].

However, questions remain concerning the safety of clinical coronary artery tissue ablation with the holmium: YAG laser, including the possibility of harmful shock wave propagation with the potential for subsequent artery dissection, and potential thermal injury to surrounding tissues which may cause thrombosis or spasm. Clinical trials of these systems should answer these questions and allow continued progress toward the goal of stand-alone laser angioplasty.

Conclusion

Laser angioplasty, regardless of the wavelength selected for tissue ablation, must still be considered an investigational approach to the recanalization of atherosclerotic coronary arteries. In evaluating the results of these initial trials, one must maintain a perspective of the goals of these early procedures. It is unrealistic to expect these prototype devices to achieve results that are superior to conventional therapy. It is axiomatic that one must walk before he can run; so it is with laser angioplasty. We must first establish that the procedure can be safely performed. Once this has been done, further catheter refinements can be made to increase the efficacy of the procedure. When it is possible for the laser to create recanalized lumens comparable to other techniques without adjunctive therapies, then and only then can a useful comparison be made.

The mystique of the laser must be divorced from the procedure. The laser is simply one of many tools available to recanalize an occluded artery. The laser recanalizes these arteries in a unique manner, which theoretically has advantages over other methods of percutaneous revascularization. One advantage of laser energy over balloons or atherectomy devices is the potential for exceedingly precise tissue removal with minimal adverse effects on the adjacent arterial structures. It is hoped that this relatively atraumatic debulking procedure may have a favorable impact on the incidence of restenosis following angioplasty.

Lasers are capable of delivering graded amounts of energy which, in theory, allow a single catheter to achieve variable sized lumens depending on the tissue absorption and fiber optic transmission characteristics of the laser wavelength. This phenomenon,

132

the ability to create lumens larger in size than the catheter itself, is potentially the most important advantage of the laser. For this variable-diameter recanalization device to achieve clinical success, a guidance system such as angioscopy or ultrasound imaging will need to be developed to guard against arterial perforation.

The near-infrared laser wavelength used in this trial, holmium: YAG (2.1 μm), is superior to the ultraviolet wavelengths generated by excimer lasers, because the transmission of the near infrared energy through optical fibers is efficient, and has the potential to deliver adequate energy through a diverging lens to create a lumen larger than the catheter itself. Excimer lasers operate in a narrow range which allows sufficient energy fluences to be transmitted through the optical fibers to ablate relatively small volumes of tissue, but which limits the maximum energy transmitted as they quickly reach the energy levels that damage the optical fibers themselves. This fact makes it unlikely that excimer laser catheters will be able to deliver sufficient energy to ablate an area significantly larger than the catheter itself. If the goal of laser recanalization continues to be the ability to create neolumens of 3.5 mm in diameter or larger, the excimer wavelengths will either require the development of new fibers or the use of extremely large and potentially dangerous fiberoptic catheters.

With the increased need to reduce costs without compromising quality of care the significant costs associated with laser angioplasty must be justified by enhanced clinical utility of these relatively expensive devices. In the final analysis, the laser angioplasty systems will have to compete with less expensive technology. Prototype laser angioplasty systems with their small catheters are not currently capable of achieving results comparable to balloon catheters or atherectomy devices for routine angioplasty. A significant investment of both time and money are still required to develop laser angioplasty systems that will allow a fair comparison with alternative devices.

Acknowledgement

The authors would like to thank Mr. Vahid Saadatmanesh and Dr. Ashit Jain for assistance in the preparation of the manuscript.

References

1. Cowley MJ, Dorros G, Kelsey SF, Van Raden M, Detre KM (1984) Emergency coronary bypass surgery after Coronary Angioplasty: The National Heart, Lung, and Blood Institute's percutaneous transluminal coronary angioplasty registry experience. Am J Cardiol 53: 22c–22c
2. Deckelbaum LI, Donaldson RF, Isner JM, Bernstein JS, Clark RH (1985) Elimination of pathologic injury associated with laser induced tissue ablation using pulsed energy delivery at low repetition rates (abstract). J Am Coll Cardiol 5: 408A
3. Esterowitz L, Hoffman C, Storm M (1986) A comparison of the erbium mid-IR laser and the short wavelength UV excimer lasers for medical applications. Proc International Conference on Lasers: 536–539
4. Forrester JS, Litvack F, Grundfest W, Mohr FW, Papaioannou T, Goldenberg T, Laundenslager J (1988) The excimer laser: Current knowledge and future prospects. J Interven Cardiol 1: 75–80
5. Holmes DR, Vlietstra RE, Smith HC, Vetrovec GW, Kent KM, Cowley JM, Faxon DP, Gruentzig AR, Kelsey SF, Detre KM, Van Raden MJ, Mock MB (1984) Restenosis after percutaneous transluminal coronary angioplasty (PTCA): A report from the PTCA registry of the National Heart, Lung, and Blood Institute. Am J Cardiol 53: 77c–81c

6. Karsch KR, Haase KK, Voelker W, Baumbach A, Mauser M, Seipel L (1990) Percutaneous coronary excimer laser angioplasty in patients with stable and unstable angina pectoris. Circulation 81: 1849–1859
7. Kopchok GE, White RA, Tabbara M, Saadatmanesh V, Peng S (1990) Holmium: YAG laser ablation of vascular tissue. Lasers Surg Med 10: 405–413
8. Leimgruber PP, Roubin GS, Hollman J, Cotsonis GA, Douglas JS, King SB, Gruentzig AR (1986) Restenosis after successful coronary angioplasty in patients with single vessel disease. Circulation 73: 710–717
9. Litvack F, Eigler NL, Margolis JR, Grundfest WS, Rothbaum D, Linnemeier T, Hestrin LB, Tsoi D, Cook SL, Drauthamer D, Goldenberg Tsvi, Laudenslager JR (1990) Percutaneous excimer laser coronary angioplasty. Am J Cardiol 66: 1027–1032
10. Macruz R, Ribeiro MP, Brum JMG, Pasqualucci A, Mnitentag J, Bozinis DG, Marques E, Jatene AD, Decourt LV, Armelin E (1985) Laser surgery in enclosed spaces: A review. Lasers Surg Med 5: 199–218
11. Parrish JA, Anderson RR, Harriet T, Paul B, Murphy GF (1983) Selective thermal effects with pulsed irradiation from lasers: From organ to organelle. Dermatology 80: 75s–80s
12. Ryan TJ, Klocke FJ, Reynolds WA (1990) Clinical competence in percutaneous transluminal coronary angioplasty. Circulation 81: 2041–2046
13. Sanborn TA, Hershman RA, Torre SR, Sherman W, Cohen M, Ambruse JA (1989) Percutaneous excimer laser coronary angioplasty. Lancet 2: 616
14. Selzer PM, Murphy-Chutorian D, Ginsburg R, Wexler L (1985) Optimizing strategies for laser angioplasty. Invest Radiol 20: 860–866
15. Spies JB, Bakal CW, Burke DR, Bonnier JJ (1990) Guidlines for percutaneous transluminal angioplasty. Radiology 177: 619–626
16. Van Gemert MC, Schets G, Stassen EG (1985) Modeling of (coronary) laser-angioplasty. Lasers Surg Med 5: 219–234
17. Van Gemert MC, Welch AJ, Bonnier JJ, Valvano JW, Yoon G, Rastegar S (1986) Some physical concepts in laser angioplasty. Sem Interven Radiol 3: 27–38
18. Welch AJ, Valvano JW, Pearce JA, Hayes LJ, Motamedi M (1985) Effect of laser radiation on tissue during laser angioplasty. Lasers Surg Med 5: 251–264
19. White CJ, Ramee SR, Mesa JE, Collins TJ, Murgo JP, Godfrey M (1990) Recanalization of totally occluded arteries using a holmium: YAG laser and lensed optical fiber (abstract). Circulation 82 (suppl III): III–677

Author's address:
C. White, M. D.
Director, Cardiac Catheterization Laboratory
Alton Ochsner Medical Foundation
1514 Jefferson Highway
New Orleans, LA 70121 USA

An Update of Peripheral Laser Angioplasty

P. A. Gaines

Department of Diagnostic Radiology, Northern General Hospital, Sheffield, England

Introduction

In the early 1980s the potential for the use of lasers to ablate atheroma was demonstrated experimentally by Macruz [31], Lee [24] and Choy [5]. The first in vivo human work appeared in 1984 [13, 15]. Early studies [7, 16, 20] with bare fibres coupled to Argon and Nd: YAG (neodymium: yttrium aluminium garnet) generators produced only a fine channel with a modest (50%) technical success rate. However, the results were associated with an unacceptable number of arterial perforations (25–30%).

Subsequent work has been directed to producing a high primary success rate with a low number of complications by modifying:
a) the delivery catheter;
b) the laser energy delivered;
c) the plaque to improve selective ablation.

Sufficient work has now been done with the more frequently used systems to assess their usefulness by comparison with conventional balloon angioplasty. This article will review these aspects of laser angioplasty.

Modifying the delivery catheter

"Hot tip" and sapphire

The initial high vascular perforation rate for the bare fibre was thought to be due to a combination of the blunt mechanical property of the fibre tip and a direct photo-thermal effect directed at a small area of vessel wall. The tip of the catheter was subsequently modified by the addition of either a 1- to 3-mm metal cap mounted on a 300-μm single fibre (laser probe or "hot tip") or a 1.8- to 3-mm sapphire lens mounted on a 600-μm fibre.

The laser probe is heated by either continuous wave argon or Nd: YAG energy to approximately 400 °C in tissue, and recanalisation produced by a combination of direct heat and the mechanical property of the shape of the tip. A subsequent modification to the laser probe allows 10% of energy to exit from the tip through a narrow window so that this hybrid probe could be guided by a lumen produced by direct laser energy [3]. The sapphire probes are usually coupled to a continuous wave Nd: YAG generator [21]. The light produced (1064 nm) is poorly absorbed by the tissues and the sapphire tip serves to focus the beam in front of the catheter, increasing the power density of the focussed spot. There is some scattering around the lens that produces a widening of the crater. Although ablation may be due to a direct photo-thermal effect, much of the damage is thought to be due to heating of a preliminary layer of carbonised tissue. The clinical results of these tip modifications will be discussed in some depth later.

The LASTAC system

Direct argon laser light has a wavelength (488 nm, 514 nm) that is preferentially absorbed by atheroma, producing tissue ablation by a direct photo-thermal effect [39]. To maintain a bare fibre centrally within the artery the LASTAC system (G V Medical, Minneapolis, USA) utilises a proximal balloon so that energy is directed coaxially down the lumen and not against the wall. A tiny lens mounted on the 200-μm fibre diverges the light to a 40° cone angle to produce a larger area of ablation 3 mm from the tip of the bare fibre. Saline is required to provide a blood-free field. The system has been used successfully to recanalize 11 of 11 superficial femoral artery (SFA) stenoses, 22 of 25 (87%) of SFA/popliteal occlusions, and 5 of 5 iliac occlusions [36].

The "Smart" system

The "Smart" laser (M C M Laboratory, California) has been developed to recognize plaque by laser-excited fluorescence spectroscopy and then selectively ablate the disease using a laser ideally tuned to atheroma. Using this system, it should be possible to recognize normal arterial wall between and underneath plaque, particularly within tortuous vessels and, therefore, hopefully reduce the perforation rate.

Laser-induced fluorescence is capable of discriminating between normal and atherosclerotic vessel wall [1, 9, 25, 26]. The "Smart" system uses a shuttered, 325-nm helium-cadmium laser source to provide the fluorescence spectra. These are analysed by a computer which then triggers the therapeutic laser. Atheroma preferentially absorbs more laser energy of wavelength 420 to 530 nm than does normal vessel wall [39]. The "Smart" system uses a flashlamp-excited dye laser tuned to 480 nm with high-energy 20-usec pulses. Both the "probe" and "treat" modalities use the same 200 um and 500 um silica fibres. Geschwind [14] has successfully treated 19 SFA occlusions with lengths between 3 to 25 cm. Leon [27] crossed 10 of 12 (83%) femoropopliteal occlusions which were balloon dilated in seven cases (58% successfully treated). Despite the use of pulsed laser energy, calcium within the plaque accounted for the failures, and those calcified lesions that were crossed required high energy. Both centres still experienced vascular perforations.

Multifibre catheters

Cothren [6], working at the Massachusetts Institute of Technology, conceived and developed the idea of a multifibre catheter, which was subsequently taken up by commercial companies. In the original model, nine optical fibres were capped by an optical shield that allowed direct contact with the target lesion. Multiple fibres allow a large crater to be produced with lower power requirements than if a solitary fibre was used. The catheters are now flexible and subsequent modifications have placed the fibres around a central channel allowing over-the-wire delivery of the catheter. The design allows fibres to be fired singly or in unison and should provide the possibility of rapid "probe" and "treat" ablation of even eccentric lesions.

Modifying the laser energy

The primary ablative mechanism of continuous wave laser is a conversion of light into heat, leading eventually to plaque vaporisation. This results histologically in a thin carbonised layer on top of a zone of protein coagulation which is surrounded by an area vacuolization [8]. The ability to vaporise using the photo-thermal mechanism depends partly upon the depth of penetration of laser energy. The further the penetration, the more the dissipation of energy and the smaller the effect. The absorption into non-coloured tissue is shown in Table 1. The strong absorption and poor penetration of Er: YAG and CO_2 laser light would be ideal but for problems inherent in transmission of the light down optical fibres. However, it does make sense to use wavelengths that are well absorbed with low penetration capable of making surgical-type incisions. Such lasers currently available are the tunable dye lasers and the excimers (excited dimers: XeCl, KrF). The high perforation of continuous wave laser angioplasty bare fibres was to an extent blamed on the thermal effect produced. Pulsed laser systems are able to deliver high peak energy pulses of sufficiently short duration and interpulse delay so as to allow diffusion of heat produced. Excimers already have high photon energy and tissue absorption because of the short wavelength. When the energy is pulsed the resultant craters produced in atheroma show little or no evidence of thermal damage, although there is debate as to whether removal of tissue is via non-thermal or thermal injury [8, 17, 34]. Theoretically, these high pulses of energy are capable of ablating calcified plaque. High-power pulses of excimer light are difficult to transmit down optical fibres, but this is possible by prolonging the pulse duration to around 150 ns [29]. Litvak [30], using a XeCl excimer laser (wavelength 308 nm, repetition rate: 20 Hz with a pulse width of 120–160 ns), treated 17 of 22 (77%) femoropopliteal occlusions, a success rate similar to conventional or "hot tip" continuous wave laser assisted angioplasty. Of note was the successful crossing of a densely calcified plaque. Similarly, Mohr [32], using a XeCl excimer has successfully treated 89% of patients who had undergone unsuccessful conventional angioplasty.

The cosmetic microscopic results from pulsed excimer laser are appealing, but there is little good evidence to suggest that this laser has any advantage over continuous-wave thermal laser therapy using the laser probe or sapphire tip. Indeed, thermal vaporisation may have long-term advantages. Experimental work has shown reduced platelet adhesion to the angioplasty site following "hot tip" ablation compared to excimer laser therapy or balloon dilatation [3, 4]. If platelet-released growth factors are the prime initiator of smooth muscle proliferation and re-stenosis, then thermal ablation without balloon dilatation (sole laser therapy) may be rewarding in reducing the re-stenosis rate. Animal work is available to support this. Sanborn [41] showed reduced re-stenosis following laser thermal angioplasty on rabbit iliac arteries compared to balloon angioplasty, and has also shown good patency in human infra-popliteal vessels [43].

Table 1. The wavelength and tissue penetration of different laser energies.

Medium	KrF	XeCl	Dye	Argon	Nd: YAG	Ho	Er: YAG	CO_2
Wavelength nm	248	308	400– 750	488/515	1 064	2 060	2 940	10 600
Penetration μm	5	25	333–2 500	500/714	1 400	286	2	20

Modifying plaque

Yellow atheroma absorbs more of wavelength 450–500 nm than normal aorta by a factor of 2 [39]. Tetracycline absorbs light in 355 nm range and selectively binds to atheroma in vitro and in vivo. When atheroma pre-treated with tetracycline is exposed to pulsed laser energy the ablation of atheroma is further increased by a factor 1.4 to 2 compared to non-treated atheroma [44]. Other chromophores have also been studied. There is selective absorption of haematoporphyrin derivative into human atheroma, and it is suggested that this may also be used to enhance laser angioplasty in a similar way that it is used for photodynamic therapy on tumours [45]. The major yellow chromophores found in atheroma are carotenes. By delivering oral beta carotene to 10 volunteers who subsequently underwent endarterectomy for carotid disease Prince [40] showed a 50-fold increase in beta carotene content of the atheroma and a four-fold increase in the absorption in 480 nm light.

Whilst this modification of plaque to increase the absorption of laser energy is interesting, it has yet to be used clinically on any significant scale.

Assessment of the value of laser angioplasty

For laser technology to be considered an advance in the percutaneous management of peripheral vascular disease, it must be compared with conventional balloon angioplasty. More specifically, comparison should encompass: a) primary success, b) long-term patency, c) safety, and d) cost.

Primary success

The data from some smaller preliminary studies have been provided earlier.

A comparative assessment is only possible for the femoro-popliteal vessels since this is where the majority of laser work has been performed. Data is now available in sufficient numbers from contact Nd: YAG laser angioplasty with sapphire tips and laser probe angioplasty. The primary success and follow-up of conventional therapy in the femoro-popliteal vessels is shown in Table 2.

The primary success rate for femoro-popliteal stenoses treated by conventional means is so high (95%) that most workers would probably not approach these with laser angioplasty unless as part of a feasibility study.

Lammer [22] approached 117 femoro-popliteal occlusions with lengths ranging from 2 to 24 cm with various sapphire-tipped contact probes, using Nd: YAG 1064 nm energy with a primary success rate following balloon dilatation of 78%. This is little different from conventional angioplasty. Sanborn [42] reports probably the largest series of 219 cases with femoro-popliteal stenoses and occlusions treated with a laser probe. Ninety-eight percent of 45 stenoses were successfully crossed. Of 174 occlusions there was an overall primary success rate of 70%, which is no better than conventional angioplasty. However, when these lesions were subdivided into those occlusions which were "suitable" for conventional therapy and those that were not, the "suitable" cases had a primary success rates of 81% and there was still a 61% primary angioplasty success rate in those cases considered "unsuitable" for conventional balloon therapy. This translates into a 56% clinical success rate for those "unsuitable" cases. Whilst this

Table 2. The reported primary success rate and long-term patency of *conventional* angioplasty. YR refers to the years of patient recruitment into the study. FON=Fontaine clinical staging.

Paper	No. Cases	Type of lesion		Primary success %	Long-term patency (years)					Ref.
					0.5	1	2	3	5	
Zeitler	140	Stenosis	(Fon.II)	91				81		34
1976–1982	73	Stenosis	(Fon.III&IV)	85				76		
	104	Occlusion <10 cm	(Fon.II)	90				78		
	88	Occlusion <10 cm	(Fo.III&IV)	73				79		
	34	Occlusion >10 cm	(Fon.II)	59				64		
	60	Occlusion >10 cm	(Fo.III&IV)	50				39		
Gallino	107	Stenoses		91			74			35
1977–1983	33	Occlusion > 3 cm		72			45			
Gailer 1983	751	Stenoses		96	86	82	76	75		36
(Multicentre)		Occlusions		86	82		72	68		
Krepel		Stenoses		83-98						
1973–1983	127	Occlusion < 3 cm		89		81	77	70	70	37
		Occlusion > 3 cm		26						
Murray	116	Stenoses		96	75	72	72	54		38
1978–1985	77	Occlusions		78	94	86	82	73		
Morgenstern	41	Occlusions 1- 4 cm		95						39
1981–1988	29	Occlusions 5-10 cm		86						

is impressive, the usefulness of being able to salvage failed conventional procedures depends upon the modern failure rate of conventional angioplasty. Morgenstern [33] provides the most contemporary conventional data (Table 2). He reports the overall success rate for treating femoropopliteal disease as 91%, which means that a contact laser probe would only be of value in 56% of those 9% failures, or only 5% of the total cases.

Comparative studies, in a single centre are uncommon. Jeans [18], in a group of 50 patients with SFA occlusions, found no significant difference in the primary success rate of laser compared to conventional angioplasty (72% vs 80%). In a study from our centre [3] 68 patients with femoro-popliteal occlusions (1 to 25 cm long) were randomised to laser or conventional treatment. No significant difference was found in the recanalisation rate (laser 82%, conventional 74%). Failures from one group then underwent treatment by the other procedure. The eventual primary success was the same in both groups (91%). The number of cases successfully salvaged by laser angioplasty when conventional treatment had failed was six cases, or 18% of routine femoropopliteal occlusions. Lammer [23], in a randomised trial, did not find any significant difference in the recanalisation rate of femoropopliteal occlusions between Nd: YAG laser, excimer laser and a conventional guide-wire. However, 50% of cases that had failed conventional means could be recanalised using a laser.

Follow-up

In the studies by Lammer [22] and Sanborn [42] patients were eventually treated by balloon dilatation following the initial laser recanalisation. If early and late re-occlusion is secondary to underlying endothelial and medial damage following balloon dilatation, as is generally thought, it would be unusual if there was a significant difference in long-term patency between laser and conventional balloon angioplasty. Lammer records a 9-month patency rate of 86%, Sanborn found a 1-year patency of 95% for stenoses and patencies for SFA occlusions of 93% (less than 3 cm long), 76% (4–7 cm long) and 58% (longer than 7 cm). Surprisingly, these are slightly higher than for conventional therapy (Fig. 2), perhaps relating to the debulking of atheroma and underlying thermal damage (see earlier). Interesting recent work on the use of sole laser therapy without balloon dilatation of infra-popliteal vessels [43] also suggests improved long-term patency. Sole laser therapy of lower limb vessels is certainly possible, and at the Northern General Hospital, Sheffield, we have recently successfully recanalised seven femoro-popliteal vessels with pulsed Holmium: YAG laser energy using three new catheters (Trimedyne Inc., Trustin, California) which did not require adjuvant balloon dilatation (Fig. 3) [11]. We are awaiting follow-up.

Complications

Lammer [22] and Sanborn [42] in the larger studies did not find a complication rate higher than that for conventional angioplasty. Although Lammer records vascular perforation in 8% of cases and dissection in 3% of cases, these are usually not clinically significant. Sanborn notes that out of 219 cases, none required urgent surgical management following the procedure.

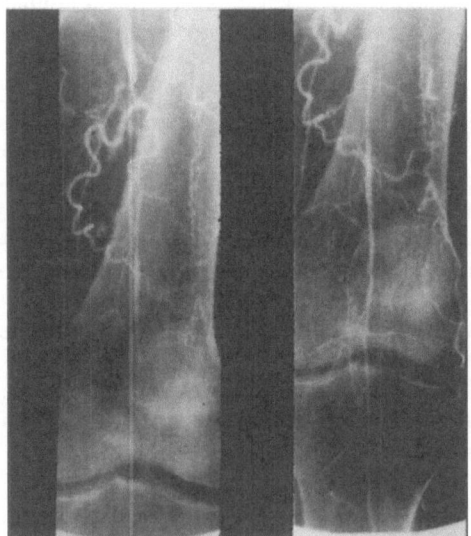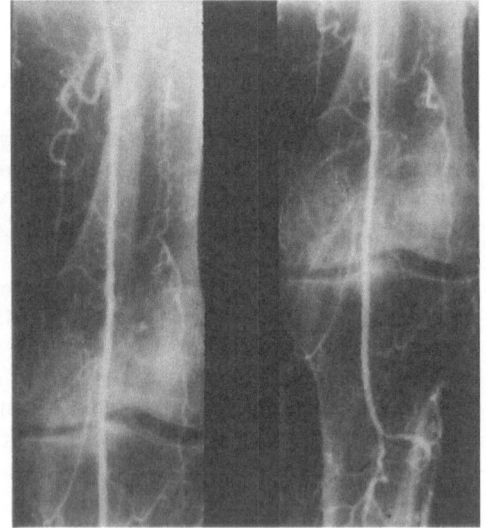

Fig. 1. *Sole laser therapy:*
A) shows a long stenosis of the popliteal artery;
B) a definitive channel has been produced without the use of balloon dilatation.

140

Cost

No complete data is available to comprehensively assess the resource implications of laser angioplasty. Levy [28] estimated in an American community hospital that to achieve primary success, laser-assisted angioplasty was 1.6 times more expensive than conventional angioplasty. In England, the differential is likely to be considerably higher than that, and in order to reap the financial benefits of treating the extra 5-18% of cases possible by laser angioplasty if used only when conventional means have failed (see earlier "Primary Success") then a high case load would be required. There are no studies evaluating the financial implications of either any improvement in long-term patency suggested by Sanborn [42], or the savings accrued by avoiding surgery in that small group of patients in whom conventional angioplasty has failed. In time, any benefits provided by lasers will need cost comparison with the mechanical rotating recanalisation devices, percutaneous atherectomy techniques and stents.

Conclusion

Laser angioplasty remains an exciting therapeutic modality as a close liason between the clinician and the commercial world. The present laser systems appear comparable and permit the successful recanalisation of arterial vascular occlusions not possible by conventional means. There are potential benefits of laser angioplasty on long-term patency but the financial implications require clarification.

References

1. Anderson PS, Gustavson A, Stenram U, Svanberg K, Svanberg S (1981) Diagnosis of arterial atherosclerosis using laser-induced fluorescence. Lasers Med Sci 2: 261-266
2. Belli A-M, Cumberland DC, Myler RK, Crew JR, Stertzer SH (1990) Peripheral arterial occlusions: Initial results from percutaneous angioplasty with a hybrid laser probe. Radiology 174: 447-449
3. Belli A-M, Cumberland DC, Procter AE (1990) Success rate of conventional guide wire versus laser recanalization with a hybrid probe in peripheral vascular occlusive disease: Results of a randomized trial (abstr). Radiology 177(P): 311
4. Borst C, Bos AN, Zwaginga JJ, Rienks R, de Groot PG, Sixma JJ (1990) Loss of blood platelet adhesion after heating native and cultured human subendothelium to 100 ° Celsius. Cardiovasc Research 24: 665-668
5. Choy DSJ, Stetzer SH, Rotterdam HZ, Sharrock N, Kamino IP (1982) Transluminal laser catheter angioplasty. Am J Cardiol 50: 1206-1208
6. Cothren RM, Hayes GB, Kramer JR, Sacks B, Kittrell C, Feld MS (1986) A multifiber catheter with an optical shield for laser angiosurgery. Lasers Life Sci 1(1): 1-12
7. Cumberland DC, Tayler DI, Procter AE (1986) Use of laser in percutaneous peripheral angioplasty. Semin Intervent Radiol 3: 65-68
8. Decklebaum LI, Isner JM, Donaldson RF (1985) Reduction of laser-induced pathologic tissue injury using pulsed energy delivery. Am J Cardiol 56: 662-671
9. Decklebaum LI, Lam JK, Cabin HS, Clubb KS, Long MB (1987) Discrimination of normal and atherosclerotic aorta by laser-induced fluorescence. Lasers Surg Med 7: 330-335
10. Gailer H, Gruntzig A, Zeitler E (1983) Late results after percutaneous transluminal angioplasty of iliac and femoropopliteal obstructive lesions - A cooperative study. In: Dotter CT et al. (eds). Percutaneous Transluminal Angioplasty. Berlin: Springer-Verlag, pp 215-218

11. Gaines PA, Cumberland DC (1991) Percutaneous Peripheral Pulsed Holmium: YAG Laser Assisted Angioplasty – Not Just a "Dotter" Effect. International Congress IV Endovascular Therapies in Vascular Disease II-2

12. Gallino A, Mahler F, Probst P, Nachbur B (1984) Percutaneous transluminal angioplasty of the arteries of the lower limbs: a 5-year follow-up. Circulation 70: 619–623

13. Geschwind H, Boussignac G, Teisseire, B (1984) Percutaneous transluminal laser angioplasty in man (letter). Lancet 7: 844

14. Geschwind HJ, Dubois-Rande J-L, Shafton E, Boussignac G, Wexman M (1989) Percutaneous pulsed laser-assisted balloon angioplasty guided by spectroscopy. Am Heart J 117: 1147–1152

15. Ginsburg R, Kim DS, Guthaner D, Toth J, Mitchell RS (1984) Salvage of an ischaemic limb by laser angioplasty. Clin Cardiol 7: 54–58

16. Ginsburg R, Wexler L, Mitchell RS, Profitt D (1985) Percutaneous transluminal angioplasty for treatment of peripheral vascular disease. Radiology 156: 619–624

17. Grundfest WS, Litvack IF, Goldenberg T (1985) Pulsed ultraviolet lasers and the potential for safe laser angioplasty. Am J Surg 150: 220–226

18. Jeans WD, Murphy P, Hughes O, Horrocks M, Baird N (1990) Randomized trial of laser-assisted passage through occluded femoro-popliteal arteries. BJR 63: 19–21

19. Krepel VM, van Andel GJ, van Erp WFM, Breslau PJ (1985) Percutaneous transluminal angioplasty of the femoro-popliteal artery: Initial and long-term results. Radiology 156: 325–328

20. Lammer J, Pilger E, Kleinert R, Ascher PW (1987) Laserangioplastie peripherer arterieller Verschlüsse. Experimentelle und klinische Ergebnisse. Fortschr Geb Roentgenstr Nuklearmed 147: 1–5

21. Lammer J, Karnel F (1988) Percutaneous transluminal laser angioplasty with contact probes. Radiology 168: 733–737

22. Lammer J, Karnel F, Pilger E, Olbert F, Schreyer H, (1989) Nd: YAG laser angioplasty with contact probes. In: Zeitler E and Seyferth W (eds). Pros and Cons in PTA and Auxiliary Methods. Berlin: Springer-Verlag, pp 68–78

23. Lammer J, Karnel F, Klein G (1990) Laser angioplasty versus conventional angioplasty: Randomized trial, Phase I (abstr). Radiology 177 (P): 102

24. Lee G, Ikeda R, Herman I (1981) The qualitative effects of laser irradiation on human atherosclerotic disease. Am Heart J 105: 885–889

25. Leon MB, Prevosti LG, Smith PD, (1987) In vivo laser-induced fluorescence plaque detection: Preliminary results in patients (abstr). Circulation 76 (supp. IV): 408

26. Leon MB, Lu DY, Prevosti LG (1988) Human arterial surface fluorescence: Atherosclerotic plaque identification and effects of laser atheroma ablation. J Am Coll Cardiol 12: 94–102

27. Leon MB, Almagor Y, Bartorelli AL (1990) Fluorescence-guided laser-assisted angioplasty in patients with femoropopliteal occlusions. Circulation 31: 143–155

28. Levy JM, Hesse SJ, Horsley WW (1989) Value of laser-assisted angioplasty in the community hospital. Radiology 170: 1017–1018

29. Litvack F, Grundfest WS, Goldenberg T (1988) Pulsed laser angioplasty: wavelength power and energy dependencies relevant to clinical application. Lasers Surg Med 8: 61–65

30. Litvack F, Grundfest WS, Adler L (1989) Percutaneous excimer-laser and excimer-laser-assisted angioplasty of the lower extremities: Results of initial clinical trial. Radiology 172: 331–335

31. Macruz R, Martins JRM, Tupinambas AS (1980) Possibilidades terapeuticas de raio laser em ateromas. Arq Bras Cardiol 11: 280–285

32. Mohr FW, Litvack F, Grundfest W, Forrester J, Kirchoff PG (1989) Excimer laser angioplasty. In: Zeitler E and Seyferth W (eds). Pros and Cons in PTA and Auxiliary Methods. Berlin: Springer-Verlag, pp. 43–51

33. Morgenstern BR, Getrajdman GI, Laffey KJ, Bixon R, Martin EC (1989) Total occlusions of the femoropopliteal artery: High technical success rate of conventional balloon angioplasty. Radiology 172: 937–940

34. Murphy-Chutorian D, Kosek J, Mok W (1985) Selective absorption of ultraviolet laser energy by human atherosclerotic plaque treated with tetracycline. Am J Cardiol 55: 1293–1297

35. Murray RR, Hewes RC, White RI Jr et al. (1987) Long-segment femoropopliteal stenoses: Is angioplasty a boon or a bust? Radiology 162: 473–476

36. Nordstrom LA, Casteneda-Zuniga WR, Young EG, Von Seggern KB (1988) Direct Argon laser exposure for recanalization of peripheral arteries: Early results. Radiology 168: 359–364

37. Nordstrom LA, Castaneda-Zuniga WR, Young EG (1989) Early clinical experience with direct Argon laser angioplasty in peripheral arteries. In: Zeitler E and Seyferth W (eds). Pros and Cons in PTA and Auxiliary Methods. Berlin: Springer-Verlag, pp 83–90

38. Prevosti LG, Lawrence JF, Leon MB (1987) Reduced surface thrombogenicity after thermal ablation of plaque (abstr). Circulation 76 (supp. IV): 408

39. Prince MR, Deutsch TF, Mathews-Roth MM, Margolis R, Parrish JA, Oseroff AR (1986) Preferential light absorption in atheromas in vitro. J Clin Invest 78: 295–302

40. Prince MR, LaMuraglia GM, MacNichol EF Jr (1988) Increased preferential absorption in human atherosclerotic plaque with oral beta carotene. Circulation 78: 338–344

41. Sanborn TA, Haudenschild CC, Garber GR, Ryan TJ, Faxon TP (1987) Angiographic and histologic consequences of laser thermal angioplasty: comparison with balloon angioplasty. Circulation 75: 1281–1286

42. Sanborn TA, Cumberland DC, Greenfield AJ (1989) Peripheral laser-assisted balloon angioplasty. Arch Surg 124: 1099–1103

43. Sanborn TA, Mitty HA, Train JS, Dan SJ (1989) Infrapopliteal and below-knee popliteal lesions: Treatment with sole laser thermal angioplasty. Radiology 172: 89–93

44. Smith TP, Cragg AH, Landas SK, Berbaum KS (1990) Plaque modification with tetracycline: Enhanced tissue ablation with the excimer laser. Radiology 174: 1009–1011

45. Spokojny AM, Serur JR, Skillman J, Spears JR (1986) Uptake of hematoporphyrin derivative by atheromatous plaques: Studies in human in vitro and rabbit in vivo. J Am Coll Cardiol 8: 387–392

46. Zeitler E, Richter E-I, Seyferth W (1983) Primary Results: Leg arteries: Femoropopliteal arteries. In: Dotter CT (eds). Percutaneous Transluminal Angioplasty. Berlin: Springer-Verlag, pp 105–114

Acknowledgement

I wish to thank Dr. D. C. Cumberland and Dr. A.-M. Belli for their help in the preparation of this article

Author's address:
P. A. Gaines MRCP FRCP
Senior Lecturer/Honorary Consultant
Department of Diagnostic Radiology
Northern General Hospital
Herries Road
Sheffield
England

Conorary Excimer Laser Angioplasty: Case Reports

A. Baumbach

Division of Cardiology, Department of Medicine, University of Tübingen, FRG

1. Stand-alone coronary excimer laser angioplasty
Sufficient angiographic result + follow up

G. M., male, 64 years

Clinical history:
Anterior non Q-wave infarction 2 weeks before angioplasty.
History of stable angina pectoris for 3 years.
Exercise treadmill test: 75 watts, severe angina pectoris, ischemic ECG changes.

Risk factor:
Hypertension.

Diagnostic angiography:
Double-vessel disease: LAD subtotal, stenosis of the I. diagonal, LCX 70% (Fig. 1a).
Left-ventricular function normal.
Target vessel: LAD.

Laser angioplasty:
10000 U heparin, 0.1 mg nitroglycerin i. c.
Xenon chloride excimer laser (Max 10; Technolas): 308 nm, 60 ns, 20 Hz.
1) Catheter 1.8 mm (Ceramoptec) (Fig. 1b).
Initial energy: 11 mJ.
Application of energy for 5/12/15/5/13/12/20 = 82 s.
Energy: 8 mJ.
Result: catheter did not pass stenosis (Fig. 1c).

2) Catheter 1.7 mm (Technolas).
Initial Energy: 8 mJ.
Application of energy: 12/12/20/10/12/18/8/10/15 = 118 s.
Energy: 6.2 mJ.
Result: no significant residual stenosis (Fig. 1d).

Control angiography on the following day:
Comparable to immediate post-intervention, 15% luminal diameter narrowing Fig. 1e).

Exercise treadmill test 7 days post intervention
(under current medication):
125 watts, no symptoms, no signs of ischemia.

Control 209 days post intervention:
No symptoms of angina pectoris since intervention.
Exercise treadmill test (under medication):
150 watts, no symptoms, no ischemia.
Angiography: still sufficient result; residual stenosis approximately 50% (Fig. 1f).

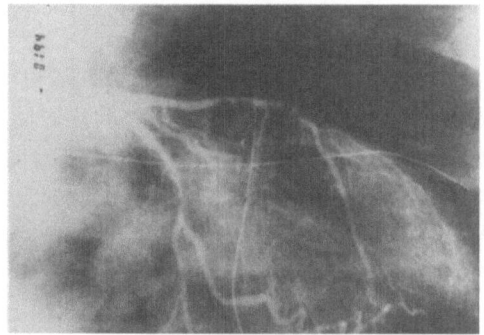

Fig. 1 a

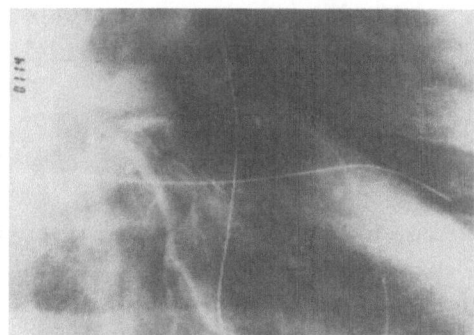

Fig. 1 b

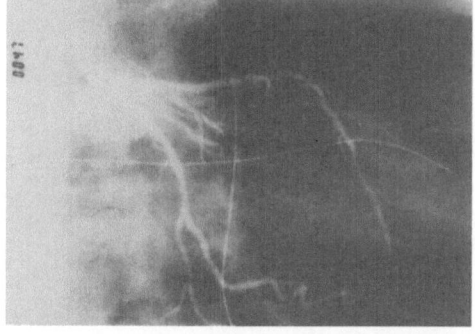

Fig. 1 c

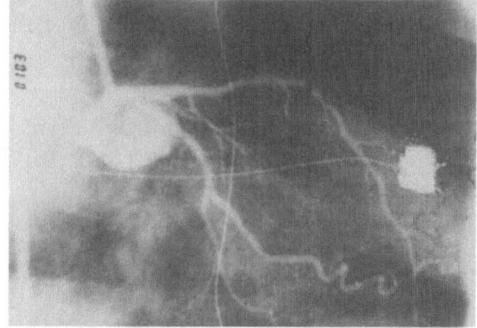

Fig. 1 d

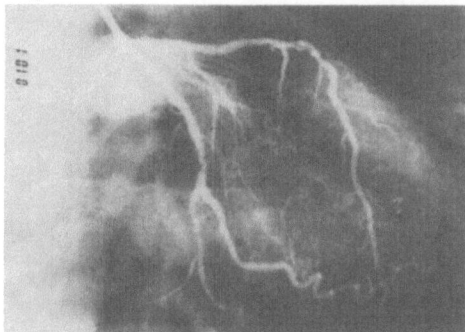

Fig. 1 e

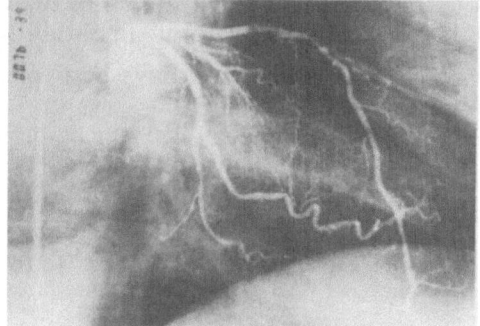

Fig. 1 f

147

2. Stand-alone coronary excimer laser angioplasty
Sufficient angiographic result

B. R., female, 42 years

Clinical history:
Stable angina pectoris.
Exercise treadmill test: 75 watts, severe angina pectoris, left bundle-branch block occurs at 25 watts.

Risk factor:
Smoked 20 cigarettes/day for 20 years.

Diagnostic angiography:
Single-vessel disease: long stenosis of the RCA (Fig. 2 a).
Left-ventricular function normal.

Laser angioplasty:
10 000 U heparin, 0.1 mg nitroglycerin i. c.
Xenon chloride excimer laser (Max 10; Technolas): 308 nm, 115 ns, 20 Hz.
Catheter 1.8 mm (Ceramoptec).
Initial energy: 16 mJ.
Complicated procedure of placing the guide wire.
Application of energy: 12*3 s=36 s.
Energy: 16 mJ.
Result: no residual stenosis (Fig. 2 b).

Control angiography on the following day:
Still excellent result without significant residual stenosis (Fig. 2 c).

Exercise treadmill test 7 days post intervention
(under current medication):
100 watts, no symptoms, left bundle-branch block occurs at 25 watts.

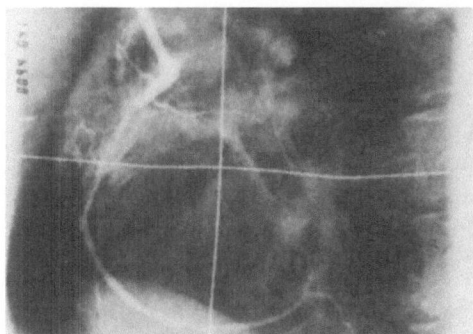

Fig. 2 a

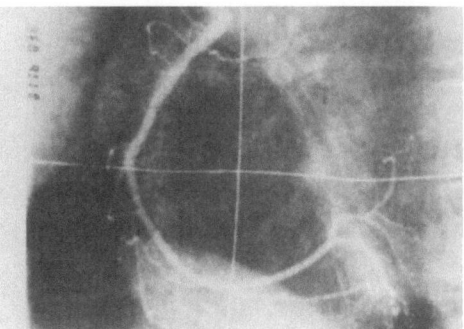

Fig. 2 b

Fig. 2 c

3. Stand-alone coronary excimer laser angioplasty
Sufficient angiographic result

W. K., male, 48 years

Clinical history:
History of angina pectoris for 5 years.
CCS 2.

Risk factor:
Hypercholesterolemia.

Diagnostic angiography:
Double-vessel disease: stenosis of the proximal LAD, stenosis of the distal RCX
(Fig. 3 a).
Left-ventricular function normal.
Target vessel: LAD.

Laser angioplasty:
10 000 U heparin, 0.1 mg nitroglycerin i. c.
Xenon chloride excimer laser (Max 10; Technolas): 308 nm, 115 ns, 20 Hz.
Catheter 1.8 mm (Technolas).
Initial energy: 18 mJ.
Application of energy: 11*3 s=33 s.
Energy: 14 mJ.
Result: 30–40% residual stenosis (Fig. 3 b).

Control angiography on the following day:
Identical to immediate post intervention angiography (Fig. 3 c).

Exercise treadmill test 7 days post intervention:
125 watts, angina pectoris, no ECG changes.

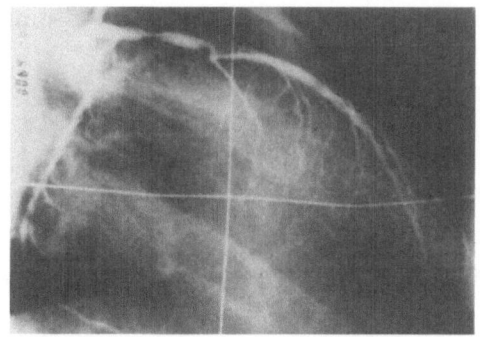

Fig. 3 a

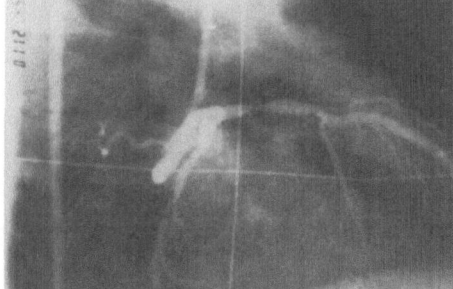

Fig. 3 b

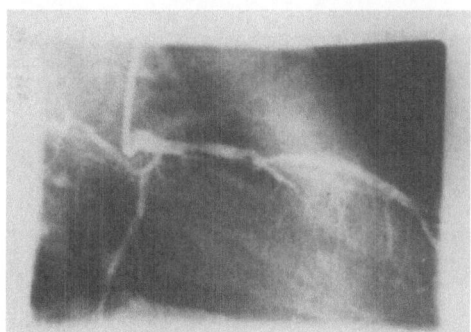

Fig. 3 c

151

4. Coronary excimer laser angioplasty and additional balloon angioplasty
Insufficient result of laser angioplasty

G. M., male, 54 years

Clinical history:
History of stable angina pectoris.
Exercise treadmill test 75 watts, angina pectoris, no significant signs of ischemia.

Risk factors:
Hypertension, hypercholesterolemia.

Diagnostic angiography:
Double-vessel disease: stenosis of the proximal LAD, 70% stenosis of the peripheral RCA (Fig. 4a).
Reduced left-ventricular function.
Target vessel: LAD.

Laser angioplasty:
10 000 U heparin, 0.1 mg nitroglycerin i.c.
Xenon chloride excimer laser (Max 10; Technolas): 308 nm, 115 ns, 20 Hz.
Catheter 1.5 mm (Ceramoptec).
Initial energy: 16 mJ.
Application of energy: 16*3 = 42 s.
Result: only minor increase in luminal diameter (Fig. 4b).
Guide wire is drawn out of the target vessel due to operator error.
Complicated procedure of replacing guide wire and catheter in the periphery of the target vessel.
Balloon angioplasty: Rx 2.5 mm, 2*4 atm, 75 s.
Result: reduced contrast opacification; residual stenosis questionable (Fig. 4c).

Control angiography on the following day:
No significant residual stenosis (Fig. 4d).

Exercise treadmill test 7 days post intervention
(under current medication):
125 watts, no symptoms, no signs of ischemia.

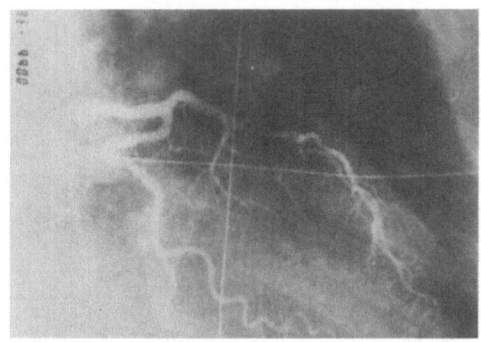

Fig. 4 a

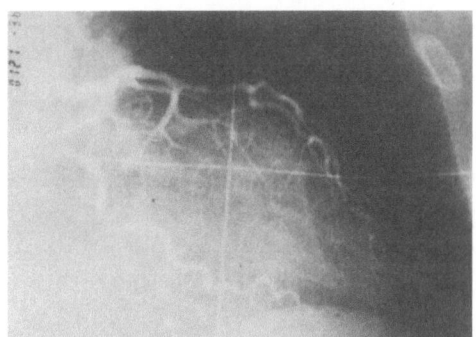

Fig. 4 b

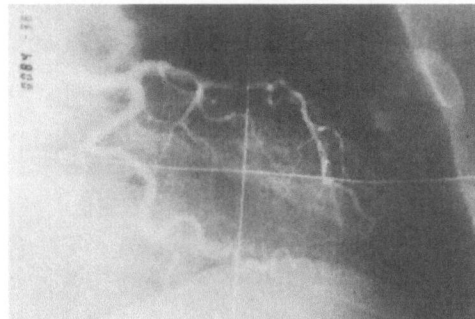

Fig. 4 c

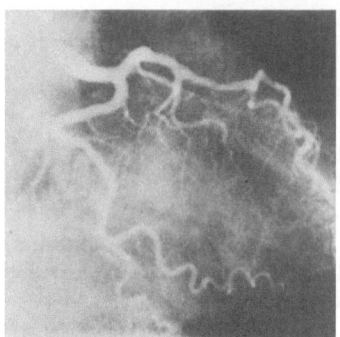

Fig. 4 d

5. Coronary excimer laser angioplasty and additional balloon angioplasty

Early occlusion required additional balloon angioplasty

G. B., female, 70 years

Clinical history:
Stable angina pectoris.
Exercise treadmill test: 50 watts, severe angina pectoris; left bundle branch block.

Risk factors:
Hypertension, hypercholesterolemia.

Diagnostic angiography:
Triple-vessel disease: LAD 95%, RX 50%, R. marg 50%; R. posterolateralis 80% (Fig. 5a).
Target vessel: LAD.

Laser angioplasty:
10 000 U heparin, 0.1 mg nitroglycerin i. c.
Xenon chloride excimer laser (Max 10; Technolas): 308 nm, 115 ns, 20 Hz.
Catheter 1.3 mm (Technolas).
Initial energy: 18 mJ.
Application of energy: 12*3 s=36 s.
Energy: 18 mJ.
Result: reduced contrast opacification; severe vessel dissection; (Fig. 5b).
Control after 2/5/10 min: unchanged.
Control after 13 min: vessel occlusion at the distal lesion site (Fig. 5c).
Balloon angioplasty 1 (2.5 mm, Rx, 8 atm, 90 s.).
Balloon 2: diffuse spasm.
Balloon 3 + Balloon 4: distal vasospasm; no significant residual stenosis at the target lesion (Fig. 5d).
45 min after intervention: one episode of ventricular fibrillation requiring D/C fibrillation.

Control angiography on the following day:
Dissection; no significant residual stenosis; no compromise of antegrade flow (Fig. 5e).

Exercise treadmill test 7 days post intervention
(under current medication):
75 watts, no symptoms, no signs of ischemia.

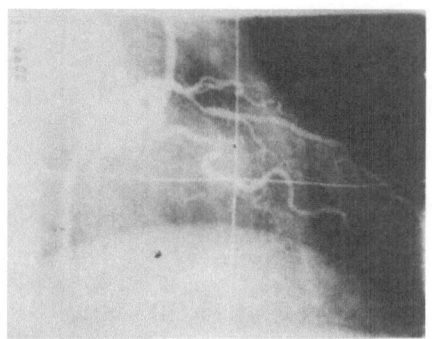

Fig. 5 a

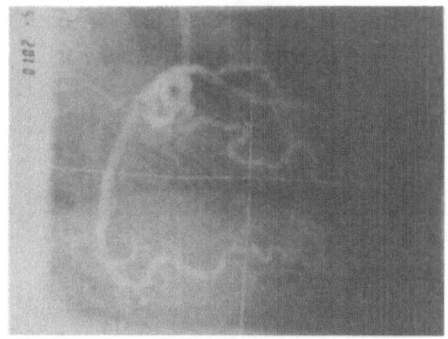

Fig. 5 b

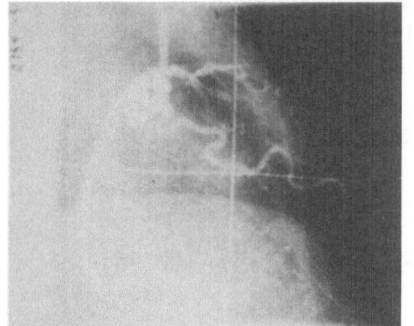

Fig. 5 c

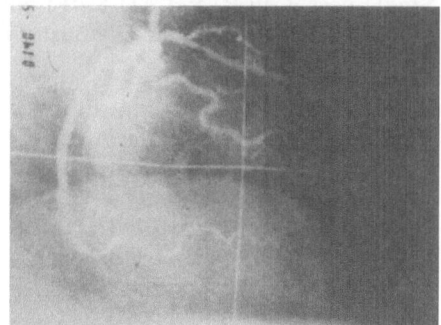

Fig. 5 d

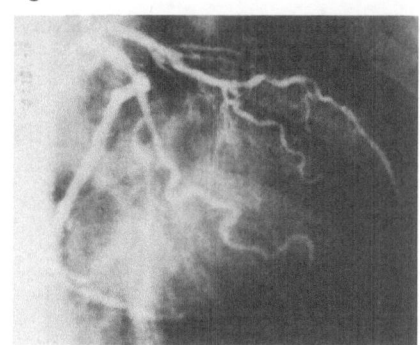

Fig. 5 e

6. Stand-alone coronary excimer laser angioplasty
Occlusion within 24 hours

G. G., male, 52 years

Clinical history:
Anterior myocardial infarction and streptokinase lysis 30 days before angioplasty.
CCS 4.

Risk factors:
Hypertension, hypercholesterolemia, smoked 20 cigarettes/day for 30 years.

Diagnostic angiography:
Single-vessel disease: LAD 80%; collateral filling of LAD via RCA (Fig. 6a).
Increased left-ventricular enddiastolic pressure (17 mmHg).

Laser angioplasty:
10000 U heparin, 0.1 mg nitroglycerin i.c.
Xenon chloride excimer laser (Max 10; Technolas): 308 nm, 60 ns, 20 Hz.
Catheter 1.6 mm (Ceramoptec).
Initial energy: 11 mJ.
Application of energy: 19*3 s=57 s.
Result: no significant residual stenosis; no dissection; no spasm (Fig. 6b).
No symptoms, no increase of CK, no changes in ECG.

Control angiography on the following day:
Vessel occlusion (Fig. 6c).
Balloon angioplasty (3.0 Simpson Roberts, 2*4 atm, 40 s) without complications.
Angiographic result: no residual stenosis (Fig. 6d).

No exercise treadmill test performed.

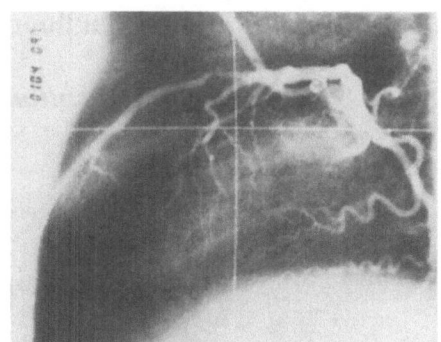

Fig. 6 a

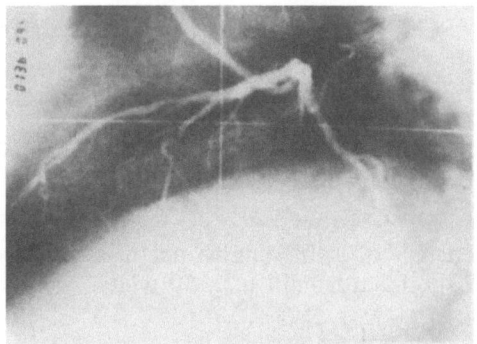

Fig. 6 b

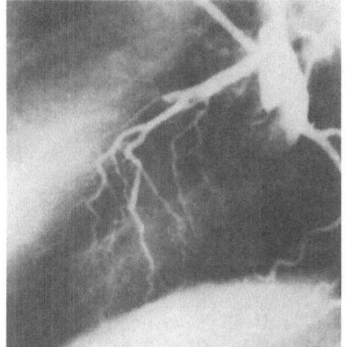

Fig. 6 c

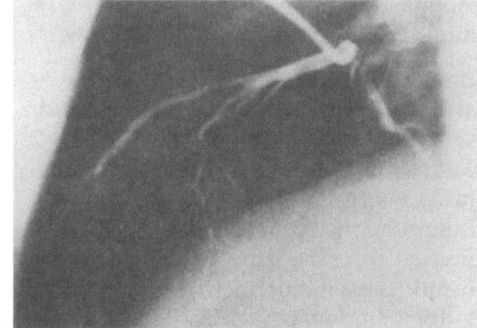

Fig. 6 d

7. Coronary excimer laser angioplasty and additional balloon angioplasty
Insufficient laser angioplasty – restenosis 195 days post intervention

E. B., female, 75 years

Clinical history:
History of stable angina pectoris for 2 years.
Exercise treadmill test: 50 watts, no signs of ischemia.

Risk factor:
Hypercholesterolemia.

Diagnostic angiography:
Single-vessel disease: LAD lesion 90% (Fig. 7 a).

Laser angioplasty:
10 000 U heparin, 0.1 mg nitroglycerin i. c.
Xenon chloride excimer laser (Max 10; Technolas): 308 nm, 60 ns, 20 Hz.
Catheter 1.3 mm (Technolas, 20 fibers).
Initial energy: 9 mJ.
Energy application: 25, 23, 3, 17, 15, 17, 6, 17, 20, 7, 20=170 s.
Energy: 0 mJ!
Result: only minor increase in lumen diameter (Fig. 7 b).
Balloon angioplasty: RCS Micro Hartzler 3.0 mm, 5 atm, 60 s.
Result: small intimal dissection; no significant residual stenosis (Fig. 7 c).

Control angiography on the following day:
Small intimal dissection, good result (Fig. 7 d).

Exercise treadmill test 7 days post intervention:
75 watts, no angina pectoris, no signs of ischemia.

Follow-up 195 days post intervention:
History of increasing symptoms of angina pectoris, starting 6 weeks after intervention.

Exercise treadmill test:
75 watts, severe angina pectoris, ischemic ECG changes.

Coronary angiography:
Restenosis of the LAD (Fig. 7 e).

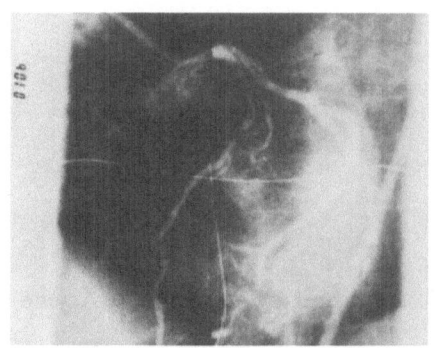

Fig. 7 a

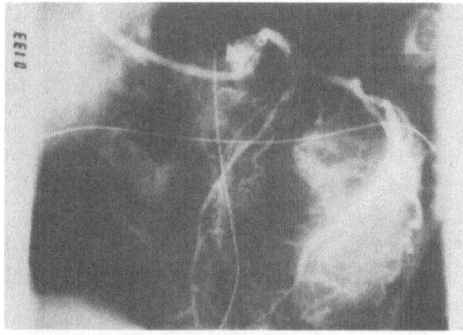

Fig. 7 b

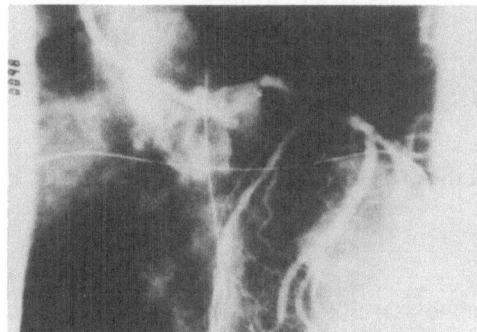

Fig. 7 c

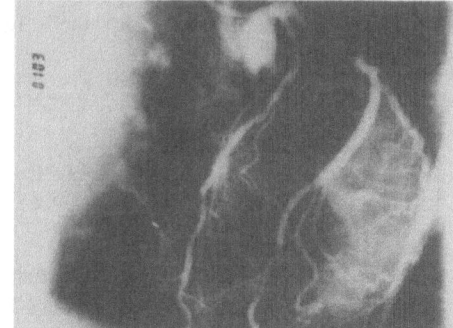

Fig. 7 d

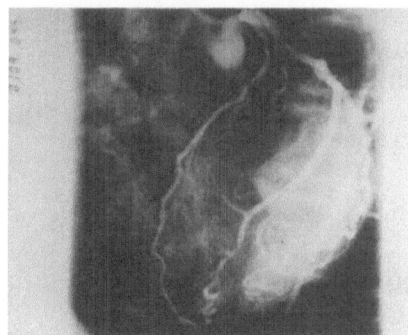

Fig. 7 e

8. Coronary excimer laser angioplasty and additional balloon angioplasty
Successful laser angioplasty followed by vasospasm and vessel occlusion

A. P., male, 55 years

Clinical history:
Anterior Q-wave infarction 22 months before angioplasty.
Angiographically documented LAD-occlusion 20 months before angioplasty. Asymptomatic for 19 months.
History of angina pectoris for 4 weeks.
Exercise treadmill test: 225 watts, no symptoms, no ECG changes.
Thallium scintigraphy: anterior ischemia.

Risk factor:
Smoked 20 cigarettes/day for 30 years, quit smoking 5 years ago.

Diagnostic angiography:
Single-vessel disease: complex LAD-lesion in the proximal vessel third, LCX and RCA without significant stenosis (Figs. 8 a, b).

Laser angioplasty:
10 000 U heparin, 0.1 mg nitroglycerin i. c.
Xenon chloride excimer laser (Max 10; Technolas): 308 nm, 115 ns, 20 Hz.
Catheter 1.8 mm (Technolas).
Initial energy: 18 mJ.
Application of energy: 30*3=90 s.
Result: insufficient stenosis reduction (Figs. 8 c, d).
Onset of vasospasm and vessel occlusion (Fig. 8 e).
Balloon angioplasty: 3.5 mm Rx, 2*4 atm.
Result: minor lumen irregularities, no significant residual lesion (Figs. 8 f, g).

Control angiography on the following day:
No significant residual lesion, small dissection, lumen irregularities suggestive of intracoronary thrombi (Figs. 8 h, i).

Exercise treadmill testing 7 days post intervention:
225 watts, no symptoms of angina pectoris, no ECG changes.

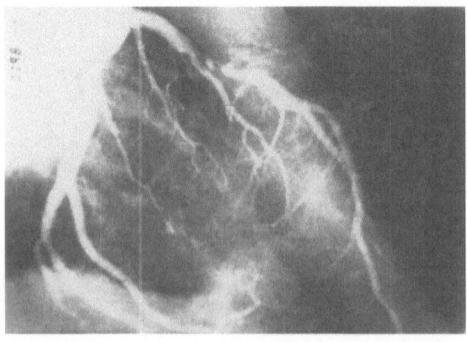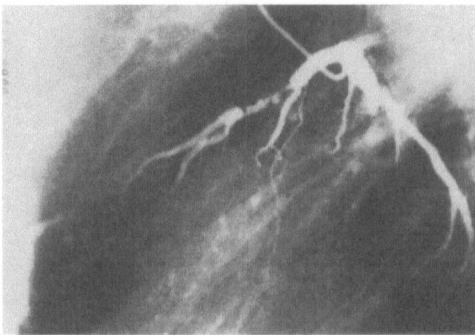

Fig. 8 a

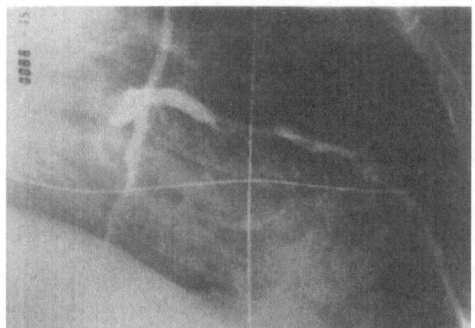

Fig. 8 c

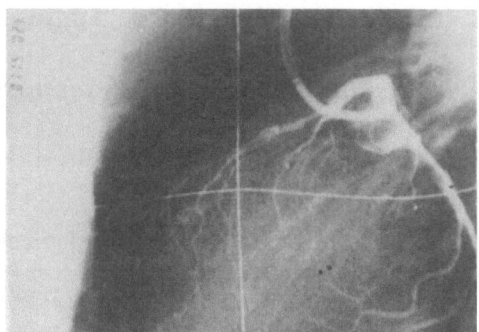

Fig. 8 d

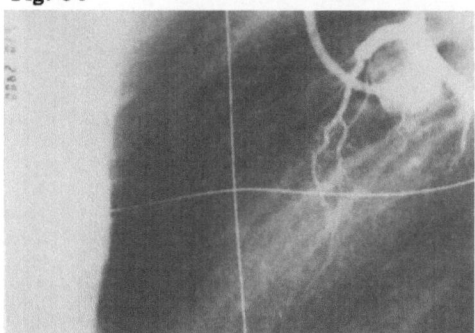

Fig. 8 e

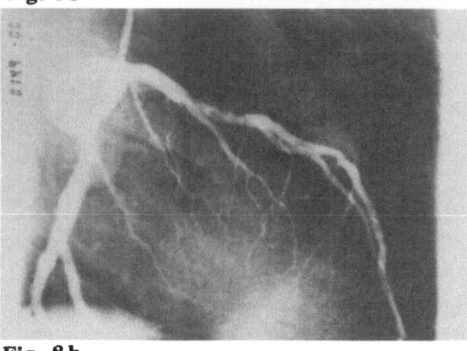

Fig. 8 f

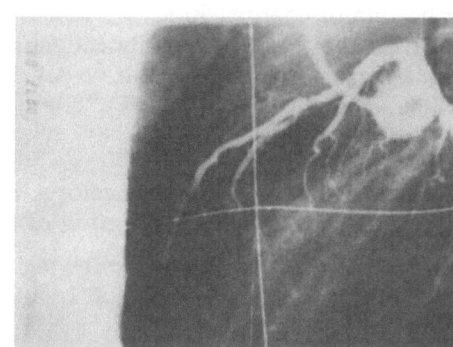

Fig. 8 g

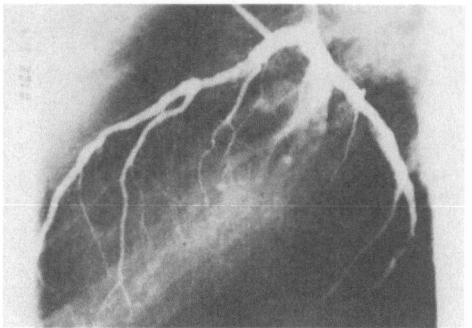

Fig. 8 h

Fig. 8 i

9. Coronary excimer laser angioplasty and additional balloon angioplasty
Dissection after laser angioplasty

J. K., male, 63 years

Clinical history:
Anteroseptal myocardial infarction 5 weeks before angioplasty.
Post-infarction angina pectoris.
Exercise treadmill test: 100 watts, dyspnea, no ECG changes.
Thallium scintigraphy: anterior ischemia.

Risk factors:
Previous smoker, mild hypercholesterolemia.

Diagnostic angiography:
Double-vessel disease: 60% stenosis of mid RCA, 80% complex lesion of the proximal LAD (Figs. 9a, b).
Target vessel: LAD.

Laser angioplasty:
10000 U heparin, 0.1 mg nitro i. c.
Xenon chloride excimer laser (CVX-300; Spectranetics): 308 nm, 135 ns, 25 Hz.
Catheter 1.7 mm (Spectranetics).
Energy fluence: 50 mJ/mm^2.
Application of energy: 50 s.
Result: patent vessel, severe dissection, no compromise of antegrade flow (Fig. 9c).
Angina pectoris and subsequent vessel occlusion.
Balloon angioplasty: 3.0 mm Rx, 8 atm up to 120 s; 4 dilatations.
Result: reduction in lesion severity, severe dissection in the distal third of the lesion (Figs. 9d, e).
Recurrent symptoms of angina pectoris, ST-segment elevation V2–4, stabilizing after sedation and intravenous application of nitroglycerin.

Control angiography on the following day:
Dissection; no significant residual lesion.

Acute anterior reinfarction 6 days following intervention.
Control angiography after 10 days: 80% stenosis of the LAD.

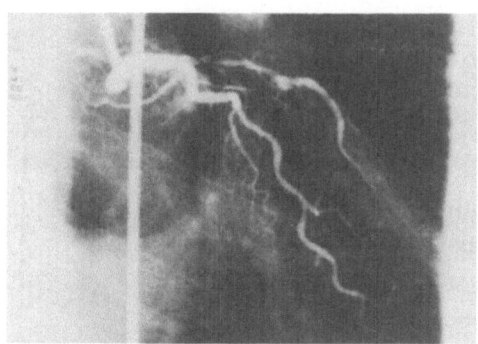

Fig. 9 a

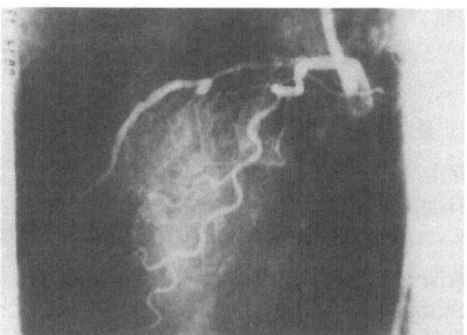

Fig. 9 b

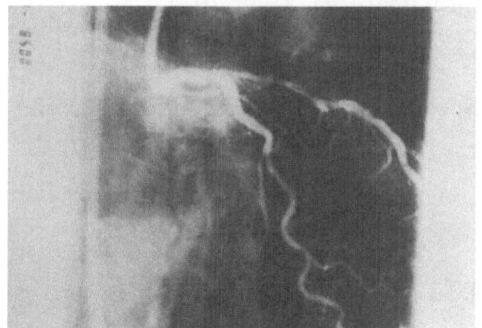

Fig. 9 c

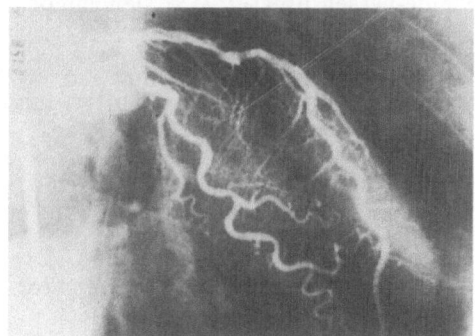

Fig. 9 d

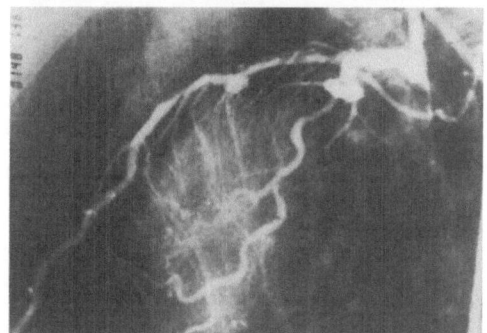

Fig. 9 e

10. Stand-alone coronary excimer laser angioplasty
Sufficient angiographic result

R. K., male, 56 years

Clinical history:
History of stable angina pectoris for 5 months.
Exercise treadmill test: 150 watts, angina pectoris, ischemic ECG changes.

Risk factors:
Smoked 20 cigarettes/day for 30 years, hypercholesterolemia.

Diagnostic angiography:
Single-vessel disease: 75% stenosis of the proximal LAD (Fig. 10a).

Laser angioplasty:
10 000 U heparin, 0.1 mg nitro i. c.
Xenon chloride excimer laser (CVX-300; Spectranetics): 308 nm, 135 ns, 25 Hz.
Catheter 1.7 mm (Spectranetics).

Energy fluence: 50 mJ/mm².
Application of energy: 35 s
Result: no residual lesion (Fig. 10b).

Control angiography on the following day:
No residual lesion (Fig. 10c).

Exercise treadmill testing 7 days post intervention:
150 watts, no symptoms of angina pectoris, no ECG-changes.

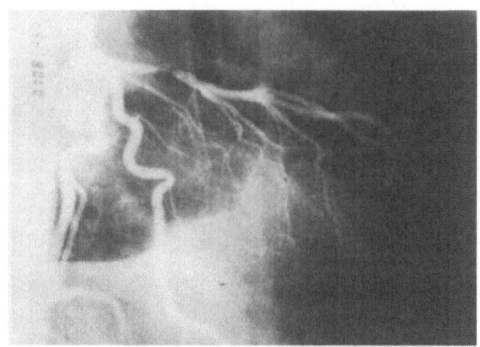

Fig. 10 a

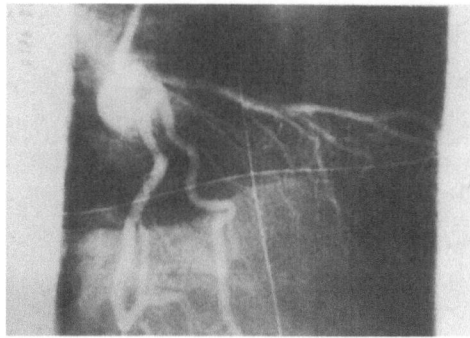

Fig. 10 b

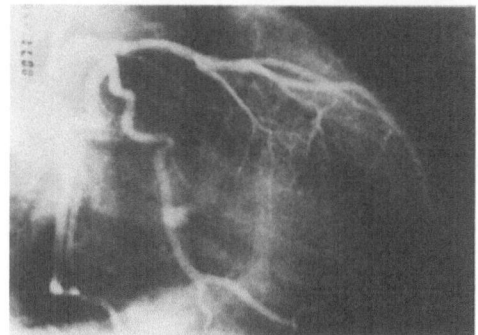

Fig. 10 c

Conorary Excimer Laser Angioplasty
"State of the Art"

K. R. Karsch, W. Voelker

Medical Clinic, Division of Cardiology, University of Tübingen, FRG

A cardiologist's dilemma

The promising horizon of transcutaneous invasive treatment of coronary artery disease performed now by cardiologists gained widespread interest and established a subfaculty of so-called Interventional Cardiologists. Atherosclerotic coronary heart disease, however, is only one of the features of a systemic and multifactorial disease which involves the arterial vascular system in general [1]. Thus, even with the advent of new and spectacular techniques like excimer laser angioplasty, the 'interventionalist' has to be aware of his limitated therapeutic capability by just cracking, burning, shaving, scraping, melting or ablating stenotic plaques in human coronary vessels [2]. All of these interventions can even induce a new local process of the disease, and that is the obscure phenomenon of restenosis. There is an obvious gap between the advanced capabilities of these different techniques in human vessels and the minimal insights which were achieved in the pathogenesis of the accelerated process of atherosclerosis which can occur after these interventions.

New techniques, however, not only produced this new clinical entity, but immediately initiated the search for basic mechanisms which might be involved in this complex process. Thus, being among those cardiologists involved in the early trials with coronary excimer laser angioplasty and by working with this fascinating technique, we were stimulated to gain more knowledge about this process of accelerated atherosclerotic disease induced by this method, and to determine some of the underlying mechanisms resulting in progression of atherosclerosis, i. e., smooth muscle cell proliferation, invasion of macrophages, and release of potent vasoconstricting and vasodilating transmitters.

Historical background of cardiovascular lasers

The term "laser angioplasty" was and is still used to draw similarities of laser interventions in peripheral and coronary arteries to the well-established technique of conventional balloon angioplasty. It has been suggested [3] to use more specific terms to improve understanding and better define the role of laser technique in the human vasculature: 1) laser recanalization and 2) laser sealing. The term laser recanalization focussed the interest on total occlusions as one of the limitations of conventional balloon angioplasty where the ability to cross the chronic occlusion is often difficult or impossible. In these situations, laser recanalization could extend the limits of percutaneous treatment to include total occlusions refractory to conventional techniques. The earliest attempts to use laser "angioplasty" for totally occluded vessels produced and unacceptable incidence of perforations [4] due to the use of bare fiberoptics with a bayonettelike mechanical effect and the difficulty to control the laser beam as it exited from the fibertip [5]. Using modified fiberoptic tips the experimental and initial clinical results in peripheral arteries were encouraging [6–8]. However, pathological studies demonstrated that the route of hot-tip recanalization typically involved creation of a false intraluminal channel rather than recreation of a true lumen [9, 10]. The use of these devices for treatment of obstructive lesions in human coronary arteries, however, was laid to rest when it was demonstrated in vitro and in vivo that heat on vascular tissue resulted in a potent vasoconstricting effect that simply could not be tolerated in coronary-caliper vessels [11].

The second term ''laser sealing'' is aiming at another limitation of balloon dilatation which is the occurrence of intimal dissection which can result in acute vessel occlusion. It was speculated that these dissections could be sealed with the vessel wall by low-level Nd: Yag laser energy emitted from a fiber with a diffusion tip inside a clear balloon catheter [12]. It has been demonstrated that intimal and medial tears after balloon angioplasty are associated with increased platelet accumulation. Thus, sealing of fractures and dissections may reduce platelet aggregation and the incidence of subsequent thrombotic occlusion and/or restenosis. However, this device may have a clinical role as a bail-out technique after complicated balloon angioplasty only. Moreover, a laser as the energy source for this low energy profile seems to be rather expensive.

The advent of the clinically useful pulsed excimer laser led to a new strategy of laser interventions. The rational of this new strategy was comparable to the aim of directional atherectomy [13, 14]. Using directional and non-directional atherectomy devices clinical trials in both peripheral and coronary arteries confirmed that percutaneous removal of plaque was possible. Wire-guided atherectomy devices opened the new horizon for intravascular application of excimer laser energy: removal of atherosclerotic tissue by transferring material from the solid to the plasma phase. Subsequent experimental studies confirmed that energy of excimer lasers could be transmitted via silica optical fibers and used to successfully ablate intravascular tissue. Feasibility of excimer laser angioplasty in peripheral and coronary arteries in humans was subsequently demonstrated, and allowed further evaluation of this technique in larger patient populations with atherosclerotic peripheral and coronary artery disease [15–18].

Current clinical transluminal interventions for treatment of coronary lesions

One of the problems which has to be addressed is the lack of a true gold standard for new interventional techniques. Neither coronary artery bypass surgery (CABG) nor percutaneous transluminal coronary angioplasty (PTCA) are true standards. However, both techniques meanwhile have established and historically determined indications [19–22]. Since PTCA is less invasive and expensive (although not necessarily less dangerous) than bypass surgery, grading of new methods is performed as an adjunct to or an alternative for PTCA. One has to bear in mind that most of these devices are still under experimental clinical investigation. Thus, the proposed grading is preliminary and needs to be updated in at least 1-year intervals.

Excimer laser coronary angioplasty is the most sophisticated technique of all new methods for percutaneous treatment. To interpret the results of this method in the present stage, an understanding of the basic mechanisms of this method is necessary. This includes the source of energy and, even more important, the principles of light

168

transmission through quartz fibers and the interaction of laser energy with atherosclerotic plaque. Although improved quality of quartz fibers during the recent 2 years has resulted in reliable energy transmission, the ablative area at the catheter tip is still limited [18, 23, 24]. Only the tissue directly in contact with the fibers within the catheter tip is affected by the energy and can be ablated [25, 26]. Since the energy profile has no effective divergence the residual catheter tip is not effective for ablation. The dead space (that is the residual space of the catheter tip without fibers) reaches 70–85% of the total catheter tip area. Thus, trespassing of a laser catheter through a tight lesion is possible by a combination of mechanical and ablative mechanisms only [27, 28]. All results of the early trials must be seen in the light of these technical limitations, i. e., the unfavorable relation of effective ablation area to dead space.

There are inherent problems in solving this dilemma. However, some of these current limitations will probably be solved within the next couple of years by fiber specialists and laser physicists. It can be expected that further improvement will considerably affect the clinical results, regarding the acute success rate. In view of the current technical limitations the cumulative results achieved in the three clinical trials are encouraging. Excimer laser angioplasty was performed successfully as a stand-alone procedure in 42–50% in the early experience. The stand-alone rate increased to 60–70% during the recent 12 months. As already alluded to, the improved stand-alone success rate seems to be primarily due to the technical advances of the new catheter system.

Analysis of the early results from three registries of excimer laser coronary angioplasty (ELCA) has shown that ELCA is a feasible and safe procedure with the option of additional PTCA [28–31]. Subsequent balloon angioplasty is necessary to complete the angiographic result or as a bail-out maneuver in patients with complications following laser angioplasty [32].

The currently available catheter devices with a diameter ranging from 1.3 mm to 2.1 mm limit the quantitative success of stand-alone excimer laser coronary angioplasty to vessels with corresponding internal diameters. It has been shown that the lumen achieved by stand-alone ELCA is strongly dependent on the employed catheter diameter [33, 34]. With increasing tip and shaft diameters flexibility of the catheters will be reduced subsequently. Especially in tortuous vessels with angulations >90°, failure of ELCA can occur due to difficulties to reach the target lesion [35]. Furthermore, severe vessel angulation can result in decreased torque control of the catheters, increasing the hazard of severe dissections. In contrast to the results of the ongoing USA trials, we saw and still see a considerable number of vessel occlusions or severe narrowings early after stand-alone ELCA [36]. The discrepancies of these observations are explained in part by the difference in the treatment protocol. The goal of our study was to avoid additional interventions if possible [28]. A reduction of >20% stenosis diameter was considered to be a sufficient result of the laser intervention, although we employed multiple passes of the laser catheter with energy delivery through the lesion to achieve the optimal result. This is in contrast to the procedure in the USA trials in which PTCA was performed routinely, even after a qualitatively sufficient result after ELCA. Furthermore, all patients were controlled by repeat visualization of the target vessel for at least 20 min after the intervention in the catheterization laboratory to detect and assess changes of vasomotion following excimer laser treatment [36].

As part of our protocol all patients underwent control angiography on the following day, because contrast opacification of the target lesion in the acute setting makes exact quantification of the severity of the residual lesion unreliable in most patients. Visualization of the lesion on the following day allowed exact qualitative and quantitative analysis of the effect of excimer laser ablation [31]. Early follow-up angiography has the additional clinical advantage to repeat the intervention if the final result is insufficient. The need for repeat intervention on the next day, however, was surprisingly low. In two patients, we found vessel occlusion following stand-alone ELCA 24 h after intervention, and both occlusions were recanalized by conventional PTCA. Thus, we feel that early follow-up angiography is a valuable tool for exact analysis of lesion morphology, but is not clinically necessary.

Extended indications for treatment of obstructive lesions by ELCA as an adjunct to conventional PTCA?

In a considerable number of our patients the angiographic result was insufficient, leading to additional PTCA. Combination of both techniques did not result in an increased risk of acute complications or increased restenosis rate (at least in this limited series of patients). The attractivity of using both methods is obvious in Type-C lesions. Primary laser ablation, especially in these cases could be used to debulk atherosclerotic material. Subsequent balloon angioplasty after primary ablation of material might then be performed with reduced risk of severe dissections and acute vessel closures. Explanations for acute complications associated with conventional balloon angioplasty leading to abrupt closure include coronary artery spasm (2%), localized thrombus (8%), and coronary dissection (34%) [37]. For the vast majority of cases a folded large intimal flap accounts for this acute vessel occlusion and represents the angiographic finding of severe dissection. To prevent or reduce overdistention of the arterial wall pretreatment by ablation of tissue is theoretically attractive. In this situation, excimer laser coronary angioplasty, however, might be considered only as a device for pretreatment rather than as bail-out device. Once severe dissection occurs that results in reduced antegrade flow and subsequent thrombosis, additional tissue ablation by the excimer laser may even lead to further deterioration due to additional injury by ablative effects and mechanical manipulations [38].

However, until larger studies in such patient populations are available, all speculations about extended indications and the use of coronary excimer laser angioplasty as an adjunct to PTCA must be considered as preliminary.

Is there a benefit from stand-alone coronary excimer laser angioplasty?

Aim of excimer laser coronary angioplasty is to 1) increase the primary success rate, and 2) reduce the restenosis rate. In view of the current results of the "technical" success rate, it can be stated that ELCA might indeed increase the acute success rate if used as an adjunct to PTCA. The term technical success rate therefore means employment of both coronary excimer laser angioplasty and PTCA for reduction of lesion severity. In view of the restenosis rate, it can be suspected that it will not be affected to any great degree [39]. Theoretically, combination of both techniques might even increase the restenosis rate by two different mechanisms of vessel injury. We have demonstrated in an animal model that the temporal sequences of smooth muscle cell proliferation following balloon angioplasty and excimer laser ablation are different and probably reflect the different mechanisms of reducing lesion severity [40, 41]. However, even after excimer laser ablation, smooth muscle cell proliferation might be stimulated, resulting in a restenotic lesion. Although the results of animal experiments cannot easily be transferred to the situation in humans, the clinical recurrence rate observed in our series substantiates the experimental results [41]. That occurrence of restenosis is probably a result directly related to the application of excimer energy, rather than due to mechanical tissue irritation by trespassing through the lesion could be demonstrated in a sham group: catheter advancement through the lesion without energy application did not result in an increased proliferation rate of smooth muscle cells [41].

However, the mechanisms leading to restenosis are complex, and there is considerable interaction within the functional compartments of platelets, endothelium, smooth muscle cells, macrophages, and immunologic phenomena [42–45]. It is well known that endothelial injury, i. e., denudation, will subsequently lead to severe lesions in hypercholesteremic rabbits, swines, and rats [46–50]. The model underlines the importance of intact endothelial lining (although transfer to the human situation is limited). In this regard, excimer laser ablation might be more destructive than balloon angioplasty since during the process of ablation endothelium will be definitely destroyed. By exposure of collagen and smooth muscle cells to full blood constituents a cascade of reactions will be started [51–53]. However, the latter will also occur by intimal dissection induced by balloon angioplasty, which might be reduced by the avoidance of overdistension using pretreatment with excimer laser coronary angioplasty.

Based on the currently available data on the incidence of angiographic restenosis following excimer laser coronary angioplasty alone, one might conclude that restenosis rate will not be decreased significantly in comparison to PTCA. Although the temporal sequence of proliferation of either intervention is somewhat different, the ultimate response of the vessel wall seems to be comparable. Thus, the primary benefit of excimer laser coronary angioplasty (at least with the current catheter technology) seems not to be reduction of restenosis rate, but rather as an additional option during the acute intervention. Conventional PTCA is limited, especially in patients with ostial and bifurcational lesions, due to the hazard of undue dissections. It has been postulated (based on very limited experience in 24 patients) that, especially in patients with medium diameter (<2.5 mm) vessels, coronary excimer laser angioplasty might be superior to other techniques. Again, until larger experience is available, this remains purely speculative.

The Achilles heel of coronary excimer laser angioplasty

It is obvious that the efficacy of coronary excimer laser angioplasty for ablation of tissue in the coronary artery is limited by catheter and fiber technology. Thus far, the most striking disadvantage of all three systems is the imbalance between ablative area and total catheter tip area. Since only tissue in direct contact to the fiber tip can be transferred from the solid to the plasma phase, and since the energy profile has no sufficient divergence to remove plaque lateral to the waveguide, the amount of tissue which can be effectively ablated is directly dependent on the area of the fibers at the tip of the catheter device. Problems of undue loss of energy due to fiber damage during treatment have been solved by better quality fibers and longer pulse durations. The relation of effective ablation area at the tip, however, cannot be solved by fibers tapered at the tip, because this ultimately results in reduced flexibility. A lens-cap system had been advocated, but was not clinically useful since mean energy density at the catheter tip was below the ablative threshold. Theoretically, it seems questionable if the problem of dead space can be solved by an increased number of fibers packed into the catheter tip. Furthermore, the cladding of the individual fiber, the shape as well as the fixation will limit this technology. Thus, the catheter device is still the true Achilles heel of excimer laser coronary angioplasty, irrespective of the system used.

What are the current options of excimer laser coronary angioplasty?

After excimer laser coronary angioplasty has been shown to be feasible and the initial overwhelming clinical expectations have been normalized, the rational analysis of the current experience can be summarized as follows: 1) Coronary excimer laser angioplasty seems to provide a mechanism for ablation of intracoronary atherosclerotic tissue which, as an adjunct to PTCA, might be especially interesting for treatment of Type-C and ostial lesions. 2) ELCA is probably not an appropriate technique for reducing the incidence of restenosis in comparison to PTCA. 3) Today, coronary excimer laser angioplasty cannot be accepted as a competetive technique to PTCA when used as a stand-alone procedure.

Laser coronary angioplasty, however, is still at its early stage: the earliest clinical trials were started only about 2 years ago. Further technical improvements of the laser source as well as the catheter devices might alter the present limitations. Controlled studies will be necessary to exactly define the clinical impact of this technique.

Perspectives

From a physicist's viewpoint there are mainly three further options for pulsed lasers: 1) The holmium laser and 2) the thulium laser, both emitting energy at a mid-infrared

Table 1. Current implications of experimental clinical trials in coronary arteries.

Method	Mechanism of stenosis reduction	Acute results (stand-alone success)	Long-term vessel patency (recurrence rate)	Possibly as adjunct to PTCA	Possible as an alternative to PTCA
Excimer laser	Ablation of tissue	60–70%	30%	1) Type-C lesions 2) Ostial lesions	No, only with further improvement of the energy delivery systems
Atherectomy	Cutting of tissue	85–90%	15–52%	1) Prox. Lad 2) Virgin lesions	No, device works with balloon angioplasty
High-speed rotablation	Microtomy of tissue	70%	?	1) Prox. Mid 1/3	?
Low-speed ablation	Mechanical and dilating effects	70%	60%	1) Total occlusions	No
Stents	Over-distension	85%	15–45%	1) Bail-out system 2) Virgin lesions	No, device works with balloon angioplasty or self expendable

wavelength. The third laser type used might be a frequency-double alexandrite laser that emits light at a wavelenght of 370 nm.

The holmium laser emits light at a wavelength of 2130 nm. The currently available systems are non-Q-switched, working with pulse durations with a range of 100–1000 μs. The ablative threshold for non-calcified tissue is above 40 J/cm² using a 200-μm fiber. For calcified lesions the ablative threshold is considerably higher. Preliminary experimental analysis of calcified and non-calcified tissue samples irradiated by holmium energy transmitted via a 800 μm silicane fiber showed considerable damage of the adjacent tissue with carbonization, vacuolization, charring off of the intimal and medial layer, and fissuring deep into the media. In in vivo experiments, we saw a high incidence of intravascular coagulation processes and thrombus formations. Based on these preliminary results, we decided not to use the holium laser in human coronary arteries, at least not in the non-Q-switched mode.

The remaining option, the thulium laser, is under experimental evaluation. The absorption coefficient for water is ideal. The energy beam of this laser has a slight divergence and the dead space problem at the catheter tip might be overcome by special angulation of the fiber tips. However, until in vitro and in vivo experiments are completed definite statements on the role of Thulium laser coronary angioplasty are not possible.

References

1. Ross R (1986) The pathogenesis of atherosclerosis – an update. N Engl J Med: 488–500
2. Waller BF (1989) Crackers, breakers, stretchers, drillers, scrapers, shavers, burners, welders and melters: the future treatment of atherosclerotic coronary artery disease? A clinical-morphological assessment. J Am Coll Cardiol 13: 969–987
3. Sanborn TA (1988) Laser Angioplasty. What has been learned from experimental studies and clinical trials? Circulation 78, 3: 769–774
4. Ginsburg R, Wexler L, Mitchell RS, Profitt D (1985) Percutaneous transluminal laser angioplasty for treatment of peripheral vascular disease. Clinical experience with 16 patients. Radiology 156: 619–624
5. Cumberland DC, Tayler DI, Procter AE (1986) Laser-assisted percutaneous angioplasty: Initial clinical experience in peripheral arteries. Clin Radiol 37: 423–428
6. Sanborn TA, Faxon DP, Haudenschild CC, Ryan TJ (1985) Experimental angioplasty: Circumferential distribution of laser thermal energy with a laser probe. J Am Coll Cardiol 5: 934–938
7. Abela GS, Normann SJ, Cohen DM, Franzini D, Feldmann RL, Crea F, Fenech A, Pepine CH, Conti CR (1985) Laser recanalization of occluded atherosclerotic arteries in vivo and in vitro. Circulation 71: 403–407
8. Choy DSJ, Stertzer SH, Myler RK, Marco J, Fourunial G (1984) Human coronary laser recanalization. Clin Cardiol 7: 377–343
9. Tobis J, Smolin M, Mallery J, Macleay L, Johnston WD, Conolly JE, Lewis G, Zuch B, Henry W, Berns M (1989) Laser-assisted thermal angioplasty in human peripheral artery occlusions: Mechanism of recanalization. J Am Coll Cardiol 13: 1547–1554
10. Gal D, Steg PG, DeJesus ST, Rongione AJ, Clarke RH, Isner JM (1987) Failure of angiography to diagnose thermal perforation complicating laser angioplasty. Am J Cardiol 60: 751–752
11. Steg PG, Gal D, Rongione AJ, DeJesus ST, Clarke RH, Isner JM (1988) Effect of argon laser irradiation on rabbit aortic smooth muscle: Evidence for endothelium-independent contraction and relaxation. Cardiovasc Res 22: 747–753
12. Spears JR (1987) Percutaneous transluminal coronary angioplasty restenosis: Potential prevention with laser balloon angioplasty. Am J Cardiol 60: 61B–64B
13. Schwarten DE, Katzen BT, Simpson JB, Cutliff WB (1988) Simpson catheter for percutaneous transluminal removal of atheroma. Am J Radiol 150: 799–801

173

14. Kaufmann UP, Garratt KN, Vliestra RE, Holmes DR Jr (1989) Coronary atherectomy. First 50 patients at the Mayo Clinic. Mayo Clin Proc 64: 747–752
15. Wollenek G, Laufer G, Grabenwoger F (1988) Percutaneous transluminal excimer laser angioplasty in total peripheral artery occlusion in man. Lasers Surg Med 8: 464–468
16. Litvack F, Grundfest W, Eigler N, Tsoi D, Goldenberg T, Laudenslager J, Forrester J (1989) Percutaneous excimer laser coronary angioplasty (letter). Lancet 2: 102–103
17. Sanborn TA, Hershman RA, Torre SR, Sherman W, Cohen M, Ambrose JA (1989) Percutaneous excimer laser coronary angioplasty (letter). Lancet 2: 616
18. Karsch KR, Haase KK, Mauser M, Ickrath O, Voelker W, Duda S (1989) Percutaneous coronary excimer laser angioplasty: Initial clinical results. Lancet 2: 247–650
19. Block PC (1985) Percutaneous transluminal coronary angioplasty: Role in the treatment of coronary artery disease. Circulation 72 (suppl V): V-161–V-165
20. Holmes DR, Vliestra RE, Smit HC, Vetrovec GW, Kent KM, Cowley MJ, Faxon DP, Grüntzig AR, Kelsey SF, Detre KM, van Raden MJ, Mock MB (1984) Restenosis after percutaneous transluminal coronary angioplasty (PTCA): A report from the PTCA Registry of the National Heart, Lung and Blood Institute. Am J Cardiol 53: 77C–81C
21. Kirklin JW, Blackstone EH, Rogers W (1985) The plights of the invasive treatment of ischemic heart disease. Reprinted with permission of the American College of Cardiology. J Am Coll Cardiol 5: 158
22. Kirklin JW, Barratt-Boyes BG (1986) Cardiac Surgery. New York, John Wiley and Sons: 140–176
23. Litvack F, Eigler NL, Margolis JR, Grundfest WS, Rothbaum D, Linnemeier T, Hestrin LB, Tsoi D, Cook SL, Krauthamer D, Goldenberg T, Laudenslager JR, Segalowitz J, Forrester JS (1990) Percutaneous excimer laser coronary angioplasty. Am J Cardiol 66: 1027–1030
24. Karsch KR, Haase KK, Wehrmann M, Hassenstein S (1990) Smooth muscle cell proliferation and restenosis after stand-alone coronary excimer laser angioplasty. J Am Coll Cardiol: – in press –
25. Srinivasan R, Leigh W (1982) Ablative photodecomposition: Action of far ultraviolet (193 nm) laser radiation on poly (ethylene terephthalate) films. J Am Chem Soc 104: 6784–6785
26. Grundfest WS, Litvack F, Forrester JS, Goldenberg T, Swan HJC, Morgenstern L, Fishbein M, McDermid S, Rider DM, Pacala TJ, Laudenslager JB (1985) Laser ablation of human atherosclerotic plaque without adjacent tissue injury. J Am Coll Cardiol 5: 929–933
27. Haase KK, Steiger E, Wehrmann M, Walz R, Karsch KR (1989) Einfluß von Laserstrahlung auf atherosklerotisch veränderte Gefäßabschnitte in Abhängigkeit von Wellenlänge und Pulsbreite. Z Kardiol 78: 701–706
28. Karsch KR, Haase KK, Voelker W, Baumbach A, Mauser M, Seipel L (1990) Percutaneous coronary excimer laser angioplasty in patients with stable and unstable angina pectoris. Acute results and incidence of restenosis during 6-month follow-up. Circulation 81: 1849–1859
29. Margolis JR, Litvack F, Grundfest W, Eigler N, Goldenberg T, Laudenslager J, Tsoi D, Wong S, Segalowitz J, Hestrin L, Rothbaum D, Linnemeier T, Helfant R, Forrestr J (1989) Excimer laser coronary angioplasty: Results of a multicenter study (abstract). Circulation 80, Suppl. II: 1989
30. Sanborn T, Alexopoulos D, Marmur JD, Badimon JJ, Badimon L, Fuster V (1989) Reduced coronary thrombosis with excimer vs thermal laser angioplasty (abstract). Circulation 80, Suppl. II: 1896
31. Karsch KR, Haase KK, Mauser M, Voelker W (1989) Initial angiographic results in ablation of atherosclerotic plaque by percutaneous coronary excimer laser angioplasty without subsequent balloon dilatation. Am J Cardiol 64: 1253–1257
32. Karsch KR, Haase KK, Mauser M, Voelker W, Baumbach A, Seipel L (1990) Perkutane koronare Excimer-Laser-Angioplastie. Herz 15: 233–240
33. Torre SR, Sanborn TA, Sharma SK, Cohen M, Ambrose JA (1990) Percutaneous coronary excimer laser angioplasty: Quantitative angiographic analysis demonstrates improved angioplasty results with larger laser catheters. (abstract) Circulation 82: III-671: 2667
34. Raizner A, Litvack F, Goldenberg T, Spencer WH, Margolis JR, Kent KM, Cummins FE, Rothbaum D, Douglas J, Haskell R, Vawter MH, Bresnahan JF, Krishnaswami V, Untereker WJ, ELCA Study Group (1990) Improved results in patients with long coronary stenoses using excimer laser angioplasty. (abstract) Circulation 82: III-671: 2666
35. Baumbach A, Haase KK, Karsch KR (1991) Usefulness of morphologic parameters in predicting the outcome of coronary excimer laser angioplasty. Am J Cardiol: – in press –

36. Baumbach A, Haase KK, Voelker W, Mauser M, Karsch KR (1991) Effects of intracoronary nitroglycerin on lumen diameter during early follow-up angiography after coronary excimer laser atherectomy. Europ Heart J 12: 726–731

37. Baim DS, Ignatius EJ (1988) Use of percutaneous transluminal coronary angioplasty: results of a current survey. Am J Cardiol 61: 3G–8G

38. Karsch KR (1990) Coronary Excimer Laser Angioplasty. Letters to the Editor. Circulation 83, 3: 1076

39. Haase KK, Mauser M, Baumbach A, Voelker W, Karsch KR (1990) Restenosis after Excimer Laser Coronary Atherectormy. (abstract) Circulation 82: III–672: 2669

40. Hanke H, Strohschneider T, Oberhoff M, Betz E, Karsch KR (1990) Time course of smooth muscle cell proliferation in the intima and media of arteries following experimental angioplasty. Circ Res 67, 3: 651–659

41. Hanke H, Haase KK, Hanke S, Oberhoff M, Hassenstein S, Betz E, Karsch KR (1991) Morphological changes and smooth muscle cell proliferation following experimental excimer laser treatment. Circulation 83: 1380–1389

42. Bernstein LR, Antoniades H, Zetter BR (1982) Migration of cultured vascular cells in response to plasma and platelet-derived factors. J Cell Sci 1982 56: 71–82

43. Ihnatowycz IO, Winocour PD, Moore S (1981) A platelet-derived factor chemotactic for rabbit smooth muscle cells in culture. Artery 9: 316–317

44. Grotendorst GR, Seppa HEJ, Kleinman HK, Maartin GR (1981) Attachment of smooth muscle cells to collagen and their migration toward platelet-derived growth factor. Proc Natl Acad Sci USA 78: 3669–3672

45. Seppa H, Grotendorst G, Seppa S, Schiffmann E, Martin G (1982) Platelet-derived growth factor is chemotactic for fibroblasts. Cell Biol Int Rep 5: 813–819

46. Baumgartner HR, Spaet TH (1970) Endothelial replacement in rabbit arteries. Fed Proc 29: 710–715

47. Stemerman M, Ross R (1972) Experimental arteriosclerosis. I. Fibrous plaque formation in primates, an electron microscopy study. J Exp Med 136: 769–789

48. Stemerman M, Spaet TH, Pitlick F, Cibtron I, Lejnieks I, Tiell ML (1977) Intimal healing: the pattern of re-endothelialization and intimal thickening. Am J Path 87: 125–142

49. Clowes AW, Reidy MA, Clowes M (1983) Kinetics of cellular proliferation after arterial injury. I. Smooth muscle growth in the absence of endothelium. Lab Invest 49: 327–333

50. Clowes AW, Clowes M, Reidy MA (1986) Kinetics of cellular proliferation after arterial injury. III. Endothelial and smooth muscle growth in chronically denuded vessels. Lab Invest 54: 295–303

51. Ross R, Glomset JA (1976) The pathogenesis of atherosclerosis. N Engl Med 295: 369–377

52. Ross R, Glomset JA (1976) The pathogenesis of atherosclerosis. N Engl J Med 295: 420–425

53. McBride W, Lange RA, Hillis LD (1988) Restenosis after successful coronary angioplasty. N Engl J Med 318: 1734–1737

Authors address:
Prof. Dr. Karl R. Karsch
Medical Clinic, Division of Cardiology
University of Tübingen
Otfried-Müller-Str. 10
7400 Tübingen, FRG

Subject Index

M. Kaltenbach, Frankfurt; R. E. Vlietstra, Lakeland, Florida
Foreword by E. Braunwald, Boston, MA

Concise Cardiology

1991. 180 pp. with 120 figures, 10 tables.
Hardcover DM 60,–
ISBN 3-7985-0864-X (Steinkopff Verlag)
ISBN 0-387-91394-7 (Springer-Verlag New York)

This volume covers the wide range of disciplines in cardiology, and it includes thorough clinical disease-recognition profiles, as well as concise descriptions of therapy methods. Special diagnostic considerations and problems in the management of cardiac and circulatory diseases are discussed, and the information is presented in a logical order. The text has practical significance for both review and for teaching, and the work emphasizes understanding of the material as opposed to just memorization.

Wide acceptance of this work has been demonstrated by the success of the first two German-language editions, authored by Martin Kaltenbach; this first English-language edition represents a cooperation with the American cardiologist R. E. Vlietstra.

Distribution in the USA and Canada through Springer-Verlag, 175 Fifth Avenue, New York, NY 10010; for other countries through your bookseller or directly from Dr. Dietrich Steinkopff Verlag, P. O. Box 11 1442, 6100 Darmstadt/FRG.

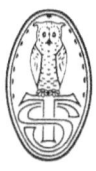 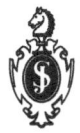

Steinkopff Verlag Darmstadt
Springer-Verlag New York